SalonOvations'
Day Spa Techniques

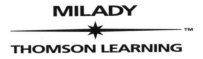

MILADY

THOMSON LEARNING

Africa • Australia • Canada • Denmark • Japan • Mexico • New Zealand • Philippines
Puerto Rico • Singapore • Spain • United Kingdom • United States

SalonOvations'
Day Spa Techniques

by
Erica T. Miller

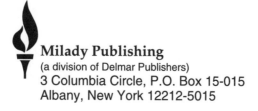

Milady Publishing
(a division of Delmar Publishers)
3 Columbia Circle, P.O. Box 15-015
Albany, New York 12212-5015

NOTICE TO THE READER

Cover Design: Suzanne McCarron
Cover Photo: Michael Dzaman

Milady Staff:
Publisher: Catherine Frangie
Acquisitions Editor: Marlene McHugh Pratt
Project Editor: Annette Downs Danaher
Production Manager: Brian Yacur
Art/Design Production Coordinator: Suzanne McCarron

Printed in the United States of America
5 6 7 8 9 10 XXX 01

For more information, contact Milady, 3 Columbia Circle, PO Box 15015, Albany, NY 12212-0515; or find us on the World Wide Web at http://www.Milady.com

Library of Congress Cataloging-in-Publication Data

Miller, Erica T.
    SalonOvations' day spa techniques / by Erica T. Miller.
        p.   cm.
    Includes bibliographical references and index.
    ISBN: 1-56253-261-8
    1. Beauty culture—United States. 2. Beauty shops—United States—Management. 3. Health resorts—United States—Management. 4. Baths—United States. 5. Hydrotherapy—United States. 6. Massage—United States. 1. SalonOvations (Firm) II. Title
TT958.M55   1996   95-22904
646.7—dc20   CIP

Contents

CHAPTER 7. *Client Preparation and Room Setup* 73

CHAPTER 8. *Body Treatments and Treatment Development* 87

Preface

For a person who has written probably four hundred or more articles on different subjects related to esthetics, you would think a book would be easy. Well, it wasn't, but it was one of the greatest challenges of my career. No matter how qualified I may have thought I was to write this book given my training and work history, I approached it with a fervor I never imagined. I was excited about writing the book because of the many requests I have had for it, but after completing the outline and rough draft of the table of contents my year of research and stress began. There was so little documentation of many subjects that I had to look into other fields for answers, such as geology to learn more about clays and muds. With no other day spa books on the market from which to glean ideas, I managed to work myself almost to death just worrying about the quality of my material. At completion I looked back and felt I could start over, add this and that, but I stopped. So with your help, input, and comments perhaps another book will be born to take up where I left off.

You may wonder why I felt qualified to write the book. Aside from being an "antique" in this business, as you will see from the typical biography included, I have a short story to tell you. I graduated from esthetics school (the Christine Shaw School of Beauty, London, England) in 1972 and was hired by the second largest cosmetic company in Japan (I spoke Japanese and was an interpreter). They put me in their research center for lack of a specific placement since I was their first foreigner in 35,000 beauty consultants. I only say this because it turned out to be one of the greatest blessings of my career. The very first project I was given was to develop the body department of a total beauty salon they were in the process of developing in Tokyo (Meguro area). I knew very little other than from my massage therapy training and had never actually done treatments on the public, much less the Japanese public. There were no books! We managed and the salon opened with everything that is popular today—Swiss shower, Scotch hose, hydrotherapy tub, figure analysis, and more. I worked on site for a couple of years before going on the teaching staff.

Many years later, I was just getting my own company, Correlations, Inc., off the ground when I had the opportunity to go to work as the beauty director for the very prestigious Neiman Marcus Greenhouse in Texas. I took that job and worked both for a couple of years, which is when I really fell in love with the spa concept. But at that time it was still predominantly within the realm of the wealthy leisure class. The growth in the last ten years has been great but so much of it has been hit and miss, with perhaps as many business failures as successes. It was and is time for a practical, generic, nonproduct text. I took up the challenge and here it now is after well over a year.

I hope it will be a useful reference for you but that you will study and research much more. Any book is only one viewpoint. I have tried to give as many options as possible, and I have attempted to stay away from any product-based procedure, which has been quite difficult because most treatments are so strongly product and procedure driven. You must work with this text, your product suppliers, and experts in the field and take all the classes you can. This is only one small part. May God richly bless you in your career and may you, in turn, give back to this great industry and to your public.

About the Author

Erica T. Miller is an internationally acclaimed educator with world-class qualifications and expertise. As a CIDESCO Diplomate and International Examiner, Ms. Miller is a founding member of NCA/CIDESCO USA, Liaison Committee Chairman for the Esthetics Equipment and Manufacturer's Alliance (EMDA) of the American Beauty Association (ABA), and has been named one of the five most prominent women in American Esthetics by *Salon News* magazine. She's listed in more than five *Who's Who in America* books, is formerly associate publisher/editor of *Aesthetics World* magazine and has authored more than three hundred articles in national publications, served as beauty director for the Neiman Marcus Greenhouse, and is the nation's most well-known expert on Shiatsu. She is a graduate of Shaw College of Beauty in London. In addition to her esthetics expertise, Miller speaks fluent Japanese, having majored in Japanese at Sophia University, Naganuma Language School, and the Simultaneous Interpreter Academy in Tokyo. She has served as an official interpreter for Japanese visitors to the United States including members of the Kyodo News Service and United Press International. As chairperson and president for Correlations, Inc., a Dallas-based full-service esthetics training and distribution company, Miller develops training programs and products for the Dallas Training Center and travels the country teaching advanced courses in a number of esthetics-related subjects.

Acknowledgments

To the reader who doesn't know the names, perhaps this page is boring. But to the author, this is the most important page because how do I properly thank all the people who contributed to the making of the book? Just as in a movie, one person really can't do it alone.

Thank you to my encouragers/readers. To Paula Dean-Ball, my business partner, friend, and patient sidekick, I thank you for helping me through this entire project; for putting up with my thoughts, my lack of time, my frustrations; and for reading the book and giving me the courage to finish it. To Christine McKinnon of Christine's Esthetics, who has been reading this manuscript and the manuscript for my Shiatsu book, I appreciate your encouragement and help. I also once again thank Mary Cathryn Wisely for all her help in obtaining photos and releases from different sources and for keeping up with slides and letters while I lost others. I must thank my other business partner, Andy Sears, who not only took up the slack while I was writing but also helped me with ideas and concepts, assisted in photography, and made me feel comfortable and safe to be away from the business. In the same vein I thank my entire staff for your support, encouragement, and patience with me.

I especially want to thank Lynn Kirkpatrick, of With Class, A Day Spa in Tyler, Texas, who made several pertinent suggestions on treatment procedures and business and who graciously allowed me to use her spa for our photo shoot.

To my old friend and client Ginny Burge, from the renowned Beautique in Houston, who provided vital input on strategy and operations as well as tremendous encouragement and support. To my new friend and very bright spa director at the Broadmoor in Colorado Springs, Marguerite Rivel. What an inspiration you have been; your comments will help our whole industry.

I so very much appreciate Milady Publishing Company for their earnest interest in the development of this book and to Brian Yacur, the production manager for flying all the way to Texas from Albany, New York, to help in the photo shoot and the direction of the art program for the book. My "boss," acquisitions editor, Marlene Pratt, and project editor Annette Downs Danaher have both been so gracious and encouraging during the computer problems, lost chapters, new ideas and additions as well as just being so supportive. I know they have a million projects but they have acted as if mine are the only books being published—what talent! I can't thank you enough.

Special thanks to the following professionals who reviewed this book:
Shelley Hess, Sunrise, Florida
Jane Kane, Kingston, New York
Ginny Burge, Houston, Texas
And finally, I thank you for choosing to purchase and read this!

Introduction _____

This book comes at a confusing time in the beauty and health industry. As the "baby boomer" begins to age, the American beauty industry must realize that our consumers want to look and feel good during their maturing process, and in so doing, any and all preventative health concepts are readily embraced. The human body is a mysterious machine that reacts to its environment in any number of ways. From the beauty and allied health industry point of view, we can treat and help a number of disorders or "dysfunctions" in the body. However, our limitations by national and state licensure, as well as controls by the Food and Drug Administration and other regulatory bodies, sometimes inhibit our progress in areas of research and development. We are often able to accomplish many improvements in the skin and body but can't document or justify the mechanism by which this happens. Beauty and health practices through the annals of history as well as practitioners' personal experience help us to understand what we might expect to accomplish, but scientific documentation is scant and most often not allowed in our field.

This book is designed to help you chart a viable, practical course in the performance of day spa treatments. The goal of this discourse is to help you treat your clients completely, from a skin standpoint to a well-being standpoint. It is not, however, a guidebook for alternative medical practice. Although from time to time medical benefits may also be mentioned, this author firmly believes that we are practitioners of beauty and well-being only.

Many of the spa treatments in this book have been around from ancient times. What's new is merely the terminology, the amalgamation of information and treatment modalities, and the idea of performing spa services in a salon or clinic type environment on a day or partial day basis.

Probably the most important thing to be kept in mind, which is also hopefully why you have purchased this book, is that the beauty and health practitioner of the future must be multi-informed, if not multitalented. Even if licensure segregates the esthetician from the massage therapist, gone are the days when the massage therapist only performs a Swedish massage on the body for one hour with no concern for the skin and ongoing care of the client. Gone are the days when the consumer goes to an esthetician for a "pampering, relaxing" facial from the forehead to the chin. Gone are the days when the nail technician or hairdresser isn't asked for spa manicures and scalp treatments. We are in the age of total body care. This is not a trend that will disappear in a couple of years. Body care is here to stay and will undoubtedly be the treatment concentration of the future.

This book may be the first of its kind on the market but it won't be the last. This book is only the beginning of a future generation of scientific body care that will encompass the whole being. Even with the extensive research and my near quarter of a century experience, I don't believe this book can cover all the opportunities and possibilities available in spa treatments. It's my goal that it lights a path for you to grow from. I don't doubt the possibilities of missing important information, special treatments, or controversies in approach. That must be expected in this inexact science. I welcome comments, additional information, and new concepts. Personally, I doubt if I'll ever be satisfied with the book because I'm constantly searching and researching for more. I hope it will encourage you to do the same.

Read, study, and perfect the day spa techniques and then go on from there and grow more. No book can be a panacea and nothing replaces the valuable training out there by schools, advanced training centers, technical videos, and manufacturers and distributors of products. Your education cannot be completed by a book. It's only your springboard. I hope you find it a helpful resource.

CHAPTER 1
History from Europe to America

OVERVIEW

Without a clear understanding of where the "spa" originated, it's difficult to understand the positioning of a "day spa." The evolution from Europe had a profound effect on America's spas, but America also took a different direction to serve the needs of the local consumer. By understanding this history, you are able to position day spa treatments more effectively for your client base.

WHY SPAS?

Life in America is stressful and everyone is acutely conscious of it. Whether through information from the media or friends, bad experiences with medicine, fear of the spiraling costs of health care, or just plain interest in taking care of oneself, the American consumer is looking for the "fountain of health and youth" and sees the potential of the spa experience as an opportunity to stay healthy and happy.

Vacation time is shorter and people are tired of the vacation residue, the days and days of overeating, laying around in the cancer-producing sun, and drinking exotic alcoholic drinks. Smoking is no longer permitted in most places and is certainly not considered the socially acceptable thing to do. People are stressed in their jobs, divorce is at an all-time high, new relationships are confused and difficult to manage, money and power are almighty goals in life for too many, and the family-centered lifestyle has all but crumbled. However, our lifestyle today is also quite conducive to a desire and quest for a healthier, more relaxed being.

One of the major solutions touted for the American consumer lies in fitness and beauty preservation. Consumer magazines constantly hail the benefits of exercise, self-training videos offer myriad home care solutions, and the variety of effective beauty-related products and services available nowadays is limitless. Even party conversations often center on health, exercise, and beauty. But the spa visit is still the optimal avenue of pursuit of health and well-being. Evidence of this spa trend toward renewed health lies in the existence of so many spa guidebooks and even travel agencies specializing in spa travel packages. The spa readily lends itself as a solution to the 1990s lifestyle and lifestyle problems.

. . . .

SPA POINT

Due to the American lifestyle changing and becoming so stress oriented, the spa concept of a vacation has mushroomed in popularity. Stress is at an all-time

high, divorce is rampant, jobs are high pressure, all of which make spas a condu-
cive environment for an escape.

. . . .

EVOLUTION OF THE SPA

The term *spa* was derived from the name of a small village near Liège, Belgium, called Spau. This was a mineral hot springs area and people would visit the area and take advantage of the waters to cure various ailments and disorders. "Taking the waters" as it was called was the fashion with the elite classes of the Roman Empire. The bathing in these special mineral waters, drinking of the waters, and in essence building vacations and social events around the hot springs was in vogue for centuries. In fact, bathing was part of the fiber of daily Roman life. Even Peter the Great visited spas to cure his ailments.

Spas continued to flourish in Europe until the outbreak of World War I. After the war, spas fell somewhat into a decline in Europe due to the almost universal nationalization of health care and interest in modern medicine. However, this wasn't to last and Europe reinstated the "cure" visits to spas. It was proven even to the satisfaction of the European medical community that there was something vital to health in the mineral hot springs and sea water spas, and popularity resurgence occurred.

Today throughout Europe, "cure" or *kur* towns exist in hot springs cities and villages where various companies send their employees for three-, five-, or seven-day visits for health maintenance. This *kur* is recognized and accepted as a viable preventative health mechanism in many countries, with Germany as a leading core country in this tradition. If you visit some of these European *kur* spas, you'll discover the seriousness of the program and attendee where most often the goal will be health restoration (curing an ailment), not just relaxation or vacation.

AMERICAN SPAS

In the transatlantic crossing to America a unique twist has taken place. Whereas cures and health rejuvenation were the goals of European spas, the American spas emerged as facilities that promoted healthy lifestyles based on exercise, fitness programs, weight loss, and beauty pampering, not on curing ailments. The early American spas such as the Neiman Marcus Greenhouse and Elizabeth Arden's Main Chance started in the early 1960s to promote the concept of a hidden retreat for the wealthy American woman who wanted to lose weight and have a lifestyle change along with serious pampering and relaxation. Thus establishments like the Greenhouse tended to concentrate heavily on the beauty and pampering side. Since the price tag for a week's stay (which was then the only option, modeled after the European spa) was normally quite high, accommodating the tastes and desires of the wealthy became the norm. As a result rumor spread by nonattending people that these facilities were, in fact, "fat farms." Unfortunately the term "fat farm" stuck for quite a while and perhaps even slowed the growth of spas in America.

Nevertheless, even to this day, the fitness emphasis of American spas is stronger than that of Europe. In the 1970s and 1980s, the spa concept grew into its own. During this time, the number of destination spas (most often connected to hotels or resorts) grew from about 30 around the country to more than 150. Now there are estimates of more than 300 spas around the country and this number is growing every day. This number will naturally escalate as more and more hotels see the amenity spa offering as one of the ways in which to compete. The growth was so great in the late 1980s that confusion and competition began to cause problems in the spa industry.

. . . .

SPA POINT

American spas are not as "cure" oriented as European spas but more fitness and beauty oriented. Many destination spas are connected to hotels or resorts.

. . . .

Types of Spas

Just defining a spa has been a trick since the industry evolved before a representative naming could be established. Now, spas are often segregated according to the property management direction, types of services offered, and general property description. And even now, not all agree upon the definitions, but probably three major categorizations exist.

RESORT SPAS
These are located on the property of a hotel, normally in a resort where other sports and activities are also offered besides the spa program itself. Spa guests and hotel guests intermingle.

AMENITY SPAS
These are similar to the resort spa concept except that the actual goal of the management is to add the spa as an amenity to the hotel. Thus the spa is not necessarily viewed as a profit center as seriously as some resort spas.

DESTINATION SPAS
This is a hotel property geared specifically to the spa guest and spa program. Outside guests are not normally part of the program. Everything is geared around the spa and its program.

OTHER SPAS
In spa guidebooks and the like spas may be further broken down into a number of categories according to the programs, such as a beauty spa, health and fitness spa, medical spa, holistic spa, and, of course, the day spa.

The Day Spa

The major spin-off of the European and American destination spa, and the topic of this book, is the day spa. Again we have difficulty defining clearly what a day spa is or should be.

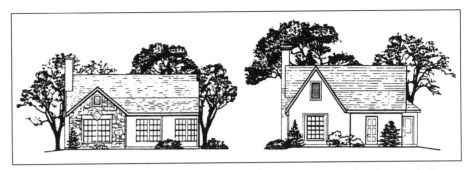

FIGURE 1-1 *The destination day spa, offering water therapy treatments and packages including facials, manicures, pedicures, hairstyling, and more.*

The first salon *cum* day spa (by the use of the term *day spa*) in America is alleged to be Noelle, A Day Spa in Stamford, Conneticut. According to Noelle De Caprio, owner/developer, her day spa came out of owning a successful, albeit stressful, salon in the early 1970s. To regroup and regenerate, Noelle would make bi-annual trips to spas in Europe. She thought they were wonderful, but since the majority of Americans couldn't or wouldn't opt for a week-long stay, why not, as Noelle stated, "offer this concept on a short day basis?" So in 1974 she used the phrase, "A Day Spa," and started by offering packages including a facial, manicure, pedicure, hairstyling, and lunch. At that time, however, she didn't base her services on water therapy as did the European spas. Due to her success and subsequent other operations and activities, people heard about Noelle's and began asking her for help in developing programs for their own salons. Since that time, Noelle has also been a day spa consultant. As the destination spa grew in popularity in the 1980s, so did the day spa, slowly and haphazardly. Both grew simultaneously and both without enough direction. By 1990, the idea of a day spa had really taken root (Figure 1-1).

Today, the direction for a professional salon is, without a doubt, the day spa. What matters now is how and what the day spa will be. The current problem that haunts us is how to educate the consumer on the differences between the salon that has invested in the expensive hydrotherapy tubs, Vichy showers, and the like and the small salon that doesn't even have a shower but calls itself a day spa because it has body treatments available, or worse yet, the salon that offers no spa services but calls itself a day spa.

. . . .

SPA POINT

The day spa is a one day or less answer to the destination or resort spa. Many professional salons will naturally evolve into day spas.

. . . .

At this time, there is no legal differentiation, but hopefully with time we can bring all day spas up to a more even level. The day spa of the future will necessarily have to become more sophisticated as the consumer demands more. In the meantime, however, perhaps the following simple designations would serve as somewhat of a guideline for the development of a day spa at all economic levels. This is not a legal description, but it may clarify what a day spa could be.

Day Spa: A salon offering various facial and body treatments but with no water facilities other than a faucet or bowl (very basic).

Day Spa (Salon): A salon offering body treatments with a shower available. Body treatments and a shower are the minimal requirements.

Full Day Spa: Any number of water-based therapies are offered in conjunction with a full complement of facial and body treatments. This may include water-based devices such as Vichy shower, hydrotherapy tub, etc.

The most significant difference between a destination or resort spa and the day spa lies in the fact that day spas are really beauty salons or esthetic clinics offering the treatment aspects of spa services, not normally the fitness and exercise aspects. And this is good because the resort/destination spas should walk hand in hand with the day spas, they don't really step on each other's toes. The American consumer should be encouraged to visit both regularly for a complete program of health, beauty, and fitness preservation.

BASIC ADVANTAGES OF A SPA STAY

- Exercise programs directed by a professional

- Change of environment, concentration on self-improvement

- Lifestyle modification guidance and practice

- Weight loss (if that's a goal)

- Relaxation

BASIC ADVANTAGES OF A DAY SPA

- Ease of regular attendance

- Local environment for ease of use

- Professional ongoing skin and body care guidance

- Controlled home care follow-up and guidance

- Conditioning progress on a regular basis

- Relaxation

· ·

SPA POINT

Among the advantages of a day spa over a destination spa are the ability to visit on a day or less basis, convenience of a local environment, and the ease of home care follow-up and guidance.

· ·

Who is the Day Spa Client?

Today the destination spa guest is generally in the upper middle class bracket, often career based, $50,000 plus annual income. The client is predominantly female, but the male segment is growing as well. The day spa client is similar but may also include a little less affluence depending on the day spa environment. However, as a general rule, spa services are currently more prevalent for the upper middle class career person along with the luxury nonworking class. Refer to *Day Spa Operations* for further information on demographics and spa development.

Synopsis

It's essential to keep in mind the fact that the day spa has evolved from a European therapy of health correction and maintenance based upon "the waters" and relaxation. The week-long stays in Europe were and are designed to encourage a big change in health. The concept of a week-long or at least multiple-day stay at a destination spa or resort are ideal for great retraining purposes. For the person who doesn't have a week or multiple days, the day spa is certainly the next best thing. The consumer may not notice the same dramatic change as a week's concentrated working visit to a spa, but the day spa advantage is the proximity for year-round activity and improvement, whereas the spa visit is once maybe twice a year. The two ideally go hand in hand.

If your client can only visit a day spa, it's important to know that the water and body treatments are viable, health enhancing, and progressive, not just for fun and relaxation. The history from Europe should be a part of the educational program on the day spa side to validate the effectiveness of treatment and the reality of progressive goals. Surely a modality that has been in existence for several thousand years and still survives must have value today. Perhaps its value today is even greater than it was back in a slower, calmer, healthier environment.

Review

1. What is the origin of the term *spa*?

2. What country in Europe is strong for "*kur*" centers?

3. What is a major difference between spas in Europe and America?

4. Name two of the American types of spas (not day spas).

5. Why are spas and day spas compatible?

CHAPTER 2
Water and Water Therapy ⸻

OVERVIEW

Water, perhaps the modern world's least appreciated resource, lies at the foundation of the day spa concept. We all know that we can't live without it, and today it's very chic to drink bottled mineral waters, but do we really understand why? I stress the word *modern* because in the history of humankind, water was not the forgotten unappreciated resource it appears to be today. Before delving into the purposes and uses of water in day spas, let's take a quick look at history and set the stage for the true importance of water.

HISTORY OF WATER USE

Hydrotherapy, according to Webster's *Tenth New Collegiate Dictionary*, is defined as "the scientific use of water in the treatment of disease." We are not using water for the treatment of disease, but the term *hydrotherapy* has become the generally accepted one for treatments incorporating water for our professional purposes.

As is well known, water has been around since the beginning of time. What you may not realize, however, is the vital role water played throughout history. Additionally, the concept of hydrotherapy is not new either. True hydrotherapy began thousands of years before Christ. Water was the true foundation of healing and curing of disease in ancient Greece. Zeus, the greatest of all the mythological Greek gods, was the father and god of rain, storm, thunder, the heaven, and the earth. Also, Asclepius, son of Apollo, was known as the god of healing. In all cases, water played an integral role in healing and wellness.

The Greeks and Romans

At the Greek temples, bathing in the rivers and massage were part of the rituals of healing. Asclepius, represented by a serpent, the symbol of living water, later was used to depict the medical insignia we know today. Hippocrates, known as the Father of Medicine, born in 460 B.C., claimed that he descended from Asclepius, and was the original homeopathic physician. He used very few medicines, opting instead for natural remedies and water therapies. Hippocrates was noted for medical cures based on the idea that drinking water was the most important factor in Greek lives. He used hot and cold baths and drinking water to fight a number of illnesses. His drugs, of which he had only a few, were used as secondary purges. He believed in fresh and sea water, compresses, spongings, drinking water, and bathing as his predominant treatment for ailments.

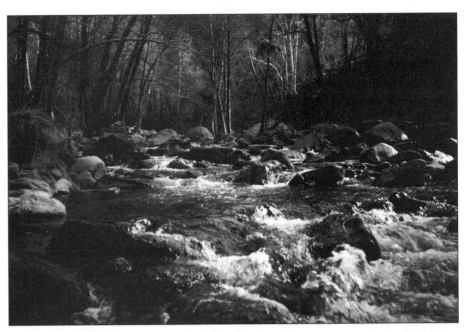

FIGURE 2-1 *Medical cures were historically based on the idea that water was essential for healthy living. The application and consumption of fresh water and seawater was the predominant treatment for ailments.*

Later the Romans came along and really perfected the art of bathing. They were particularly interested in seawater and running water. They developed vast systems of cisterns and aqueducts to transport fresh water to the people. Some of the finest examples of Roman cisterns are still found in Carthage, a city of magnificent springs. In Rome alone there were more than eight hundred public baths constructed. According to Pliny, Rome was without a physician for more than six hundred years, a comment credited to the healing capabilities of the waters.

Then came the physician, Galen, who became famous for his ability to cure consumption. His philosophy was founded in the continued belief in water containing sunlight and oxygen (Figure 2-1).

His well-known treatment consisted of baths, drinking pure water, fresh air, moderate diet, and exercise.

Biblical References

Let's not forget that the Bible has more than fifty-two references to water in the Old and New Testaments. For example, John 3:5 states "Jesus answered, 'Truly, truly I say to you, unless one is born of water and the Spirit, he cannot enter into the kingdom of God.'" Biblical representations of water infer purity and innocence, and the use of the term *living water* referred to new life through the spirit after salvation. Baptism, a word meaning purification, came from the time of Christ and consisted of three immersions in living water. Hippocrates, Galen, and Christ all insisted upon the use of water for healing and renewal. The term *living water* also came to mean water containing sunlight and oxygen.

Another more modern link to the primitive church was the famous John Wesley, who insisted on total immersion for baptism. In many of his sermons he was said to have been able to cure blindness, asthma, shingles, cancers, and other diseases through cold bathing. In 1702, Dr. John Floyer published a book entitled *The History of Cold Bathing Both Ancient and Modern* in which he stressed the curative value of drinking cold water before bathing in cold water, and then drinking it again after. Later he added warm water bathing for greater effectiveness.

Modern Beginnings

Another well-known physician in England at the time, Dr. Erasmus Darwin, father of Charles Darwin, reported great results with water therapy as well, and even treated his own son with it. Strangely enough, bathing soon fell into disrepute in England, but in the United States the famous statesman and philosopher Benjamin Franklin pioneered our own custom of bathing and encouraged swimming as one of the most healthful and agreeable exercises in the world. In his latter years of ill health, he is known to have taken a warm bath several times a day.

But the real development of the bath and spa originated by accident between 1829 and 1842 in the Austro-Hungarian Empire by a simple farmer named Vincent Priessnitz. He first cured his own farm animals in the adjacent stream and then was able to cure a personal rib injury when he was accidentally run over by a cart. His use of water in this recovery catapulted him into the development of an entire system of using water in bathings as well as with cool and warm compresses. His successes didn't go unnoticed and he was eventually taken to court as a quack healer, but he won his case and became protected by the crown. As a result of this, healing establishments began springing up all over under his direction and he's said to have cured more than seven thousand persons, mostly intellectuals from all over Europe. This included a number of well-respected physicians who became sold on his concepts. Priessnitz didn't document his procedures in writing so his fame was somewhat stifled.

About the same time a German man, Sebastian Kneipp, born in 1821 in Bavaria, got involved in water cures for his own health problems. He was a priest with a number of illnesses who heard about Priessnitz and decided to try his cold water dip techniques. Determined to strengthen himself, he began a daily routine of icy plunges in the middle of cold winter Bavaria and discovered tremendous stamina, energy, and strength return. He added some concepts to Priessnitz's techniques. He was quite a herbalist and left a legacy of herbal therapeutics along with the water therapy. He became the foremost authority on water and herbal bathing and drinks. He is well known for using hay flower or oat straw for detoxification purposes. He was particularly effective with children and developed the wet "nightshirt," a healing technique in which salt or hay flower was added to water into which shirts were dipped then worn for a number of remedies. Since Kneipp, we have had a long retinue of enforcers of the value of water-based therapy.

Due to Priessnitz and Kneipp, water therapy became a very basic and normal method of treating people all over Europe. The development of spas came from this healing concept in areas near special natural springs and pure water and developed into healing-oriented resorts. All over Germany and other countries, corporations still send employees to spa towns for week-long cures. This is part of the preventative and curative healing consciousness of Europeans.

WATER AND ITS USES

We've already touched on the healing properties of water as used throughout history. An interesting point to note was the historical use of surface water rather than deep water. It is believed that surface water, if clean and pure, of course, contains a great deal of oxygen and nitrogen and little carbon dioxide (Figure 2-2). The beauty of increased oxygen and nitrogen is that they provide the body with self-healing improvement and actually activates the body's own mechanisms. This may be one reason water was used so much in the past as a natural healing agent. Water, whether used in warm, hot, cool, or cold form, provides additional stimulating and calming actions on the body and skin.

Aside from bathing, water should be consumed in large quantities. Some believe that due to the saline content of water in our bodies, the addition of salt water to our system is healing and nourishing. Aside from obvious medical benefits such as to reduce fever, to be a diuretic, to treat certain injuries and burns, or to relieve pain, we use water therapeutically in a salon or spa environment for relaxation, moisturization, stimulation of the entire system, relief of discomfort and achiness, to relieve thirst, and for local

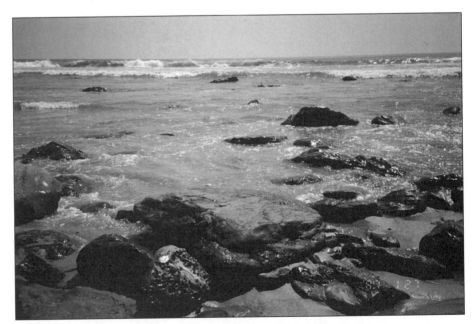

FIGURE 2-2 *Water and its elements have long been associated with healing.*

heating, cooling, and friction purposes. We use water-based treatments to facilitate the absorption of nutrients in beauty products and cosmetics and to stimulate the body's metabolism to help break down fats and toxins so that the body can rid itself of unwanted toxins and wastes. So many healthful and beautifying effects result from the myriad uses of water in beauty-related treatments. We will also discuss drinking water, compresses for different purposes, baths and showers at home, and exercising in water for increased mobility. In the salon environment, a number of energizing and revitalizing treatments are provided by water.

As we begin to proceed to the spa environment and discuss the many uses of water, specifics will be given on water and its various applications. In each and every case, there will be some overlap as the benefits of water in general are added to specific modalities. It's pertinent at this point to mention two important facets of water and water therapy.

Water By Itself

Whether fresh water or seawater, water by itself has beneficial effects on the body (Figure 2-3). Consider for a moment how you feel after a quick morning dip in the pool. Don't you feel invigorated and ready to go? If you don't have a pool, how do you feel after a quick shower? When taken first thing in the morning, you'll find it refreshing and awakening. Or how about a swim in the ocean? Not only will you normally feel refreshed and energized, your appetite is improved and the body feels less stress. From the obvious cures of Sebastian Kneipp that have become so famous to the history of bathing from more than four thousand years ago, there must be something valuable and healthful to water all by itself.

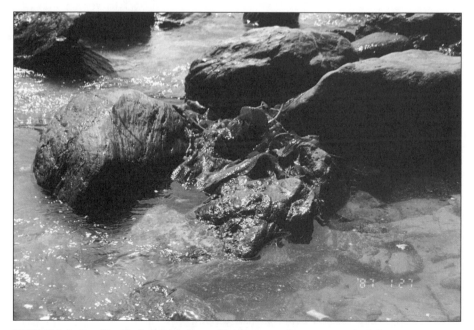

FIGURE 2-3 *Consider the beneficial effects of fresh water and seawater on the body. Water, including additives such as mud and seaweed, can greatly enhance the human body both physiologically and psychologically.*

Water Therapy

Water is used in conjunction with various additives, from salts to seaweed to mud and essential oils. Now we move to a greater sophistication of treatment and effects on the body. Even though the benefits to the human organism overlap somewhat, these additives greatly enhance the physiological as well as psychological benefits to the human being.

. . . .

SPA POINT

Water all by itself has tremendous beneficial effects on the human organism. Additives such as seaweed, mud, and essential oils enhance that simple and natural benefit in myriad ways.

. . . .

Now let's look at water in a little more depth.

Circulation

The blood circulation is directly affected by water in a number of ways, the predominant one being the use of warm or cold water to effect an increase or decrease in the circulation of a specific area of the body. Most hydrotherapy treatments concentrate on the effects to the circulatory system. Warm or hot water causes a vasodilation of the capillaries that often facilitates the distribution of nutrition and oxygen to all the organs and tissues. Cool or cold water causes the opposite, vasoconstriction or contraction of the capillaries. This helps in quick stimulation to the system and reduction of edema (swelling).

The person who made the combination of warm and cool water alternating therapy popular was Sebastian Kneipp. This is the basis of all his treatment principles. (This will be more fully developed in another chapter.) As an example, cold water can be invigorating whereas warm water is relaxing. I'm sure the reader will relate to the relative health and stamina of the well-known actress Katharine Hepburn, who is famous at her advanced age for taking long swims daily year-round in the ocean off the coast next to her home. She personally credits her vim and vigor to the cold water.

WARM TO HOT WATER

- High temperature water has a strong anti-inflammatory and anti-infectious action.

- Warm water relaxes the body.

- Warm water increases blood flow.

- The heat induces perspiration, thus the elimination of toxins.

- Warm to hot water reduces pain and discomfort.

- Warm water relaxes muscles and the entire body.

- Warm to hot water can induce fatigue through muscle and system relaxation.

- Warm to hot water increases circulation, making product penetration more effective.

COOL TO COLD WATER

- Cold water has great effects on our lungs, heart, skin, and brain.

- Cool to cold water is invigorating and stimulating and adds tone.

- Cold causes the capillaries to contract to assist in reducing swelling.

- Cold water for a short time has a tonic effect on the body; for an extended time it depresses the body.

- Cold water increases the body's own resistance to disease.

- Cold water sometimes reduces pain.

- Cold water stimulates maintenance of skin elasticity.

- In some cold water treatments, the skin releases histamines that work to reduce the tendency to allergic reactions.

- Cool water can relieve headaches.

- Cold water stimulates nerve endings, which in turn increases circulation making the skin more absorptive of applied substances.

Movement and Exercise in Water

There is another important aspect of water we must consider in addition to its effects on circulation. Physical therapy in water as well as water aerobics have been popular for some time. Although this does not come directly under the subject of day spa treatments, it's important to consider that the reason for the popularity lies in the relative density of the human body in water. The fact is that when a body is immersed in a fluid, such as water, it experiences buoyancy in equal proportion to the amount of water displaced. In simple terms, the density and resistance in water make the human body float, exercise, and move muscles better. When you add salt as in the Dead Sea, the body really becomes buoyant and can float effortlessly. Also, the turbulence in water such as water pressure from a hose or air jets in a hydrotherapy tub allow the body to exercise without exertion. This is why water is so great for persons recuperating from injuries or patients with muscle atrophy. Because of the water resistance or friction, much greater exercise can be accomplished than on land. This will be very valuable when we discuss topics such as cellulite treatments and increasing circulation. Additionally, the thermal action of warm water relaxes muscles and improves overall body mobility. Cold water shocks and invigorates muscle activity as well.

· ·

SPA POINT

Warm to hot and cool to cold water affect the body in more ways than we normally think. Just consider the many ways in which any hydrotherapy treatment can promote a sense of relaxation and well-being. The relaxation from warm water and invigoration from cold water alone serve to make our day spa treatments helpful to the busy client today.

· ·

Synopsis

In coming chapters you will learn more about how the blending and overlapping of warm and cool water, with and without additives, are used in a variety of ways for similar and different effects. The myriad additives and treatments used in conjunction with water makes our work exciting and challenging. For the novice it may seem complicated and confusing, but remember that much of this therapy has been handed down from sources around the world over a duration of four thousand plus years so it would be impossible to know and understand every combination in one mere lifetime. The beauty for the professional lies in the ability to understand general principles and then to experiment and grow experientially on a daily basis.

Water and its various applications will be discussed in several different chapters. Alternating hot and cold will be used for a variety of effects. Additives and concepts of aromatherapy and herbal therapies will further add to the effectiveness of day spa treatments. However, as with all aspects of beauty and health care, water therapy, aromatherapy, and the like are an inexact science. We are limited not only by the general lack of scientific data, but also by the constraints of our license. As is reiterated so often throughout the book, the application of water and additives is for beauty and health maintenance only. Aspects of healing and curative benefits are certainly a large part of the actual results, but that is not our purpose or goal. Any references to medical or curative benefits are for your professional information only and are not to be transferred into practice.

. . . .

SPA POINT

It has taken more than four thousand years and every country in the world to develop water and treatment concepts. It is therefore impossible for the practitioner to learn all of them in the scope of one book or one lifetime. Your expertise will come with time and experience. And in the meantime, even the simplest of treatments will work wonders in beauty and health maintenance, not to mention client satisfaction.

. . . .

Review

1. In your opinion, how does history help us understand the benefits of spa water treatments?

2. When did hydrotherapy begin?

3. What did Hippocrates have to do with water as a therapy?

4. Who was Sebastian Kneipp?

5. Is plain water a therapy?

6. How do additives help water therapies?

7. Name some effects of warm and cool water on the body.

CHAPTER 3
Baths and Bathing

OVERVIEW

In some respects, this chapter will be the highlight of the entire book, because as we have seen from a brief look at the history of water therapy, bathing becomes the central core of all applications of water as a therapy. For a more in depth look at the history of water and bathing, you may want to refer to the book, *Taking the Waters, Spirit*Art*Sensuality*, by Alev Lytle Croutier (see bibliography). This book takes you from references in mythology through history to the destination spas of the world.

BATHING HISTORY

Quickly, however, we'll review history a bit. Bathing goes back to the Nile River, the cradle of civilization. If you remember Alexandria, under the Ptolemies, there were more than four thousand public baths for a population of under 250,000 people. The Egyptians were also famous for collecting rain water and bathing in that for health purposes.

The Greeks and Romans

The Greeks were also known for bathing. Remember the emphasis on physical fitness and body development? Bathing was a natural part of daily activity after physical exercise and this was revered above intellectual pursuits. In fact many of the bathing centers also contained on-site gymnasiums. The Greeks are believed to be the people who first utilized hot water and a form of exfoliation using a strigil, a curved metal instrument used to scrape the body in the baths.

The Roman baths were, as previously stated, the real social centers of society, comprising much more than just baths. Roman emperors were known to have spent days at a time in the baths, entering the water as many as six to eight times a day. Even the populace were known to have bathed multiple times a day. Roman baths were called *thermae*, and the communal part of the bath centers were called *balnea*. Some of these terms have become the name of various therapies. According to *Taking the Waters*, "in Rome around 312 B.C. there were over 750 million liters of water in 13 aqueducts for Rome's 1352 public fountains, 11 Imperial Thermae, and 926 public baths." One of the most famous *thermae* was the Diocletian Bath that accommodated more than six thousand people at a time. Both Greek and Roman alike celebrated the beauty and health of the body.

The Middle East and India

In Israel, the Jordan River was considered to be the foundation of Christianity. There is an interesting reference in 2 Kings 5:10 (NAS) that states, "And Elisha sent a messenger to him saying, 'Go and wash in the Jordan seven times, and your flesh shall be restored to you and you shall be clean,'" referring to the bathing, cleansing, and purification of water in that society as well as the Christian importance of baptism in the Jordan. Today we still celebrate the value and healing powers of the Dead Sea.

The Hindu rites in India along the Ganges River, the steam baths of the Turks, and most other Middle Eastern cultures also have long important histories related to bathing.

Japan

And moving to another part of the world, the Japanese have often been considered the world's cleanest people. To the Japanese, bathing was much more than just a cleansing procedure; it was and is the spirit of cleansing the mind and renewing the self. In Japan baths were religious rites called *yuami* and *misogi*, being an essential element of the Shinto religion (the Japanese national religion practiced in conjunction with Buddhism from China and India) for more than two thousand years.

Interestingly enough, there has been very little change in bathing customs until quite recently. Modern Japanese don't specifically think of bathing as a religious act, but the relaxation is certainly spiritually appreciated and a visit to a hot springs resort (called *onsen*) or special bath resort is a highly prized vacation.

Looking back at history, there were as many as twenty thousand bathhouses throughout the country. In recent times, the number of public bathhouses has dwindled to less than twelve thousand due in part to the addition of private baths in most homes and to the cost of operating the public bath (called *sento*). Approximately two thousand bathhouses remain in Tokyo, but that number is dwindling quickly. As the popularity of day spas and health consciousness grows, however, it is believed that there will be a revival in public bathing. There will be quite a bit of modernization that is way ahead of America in some respects. Today in Japan, the bathing custom of cleaning the body outside the tub and then soaking for fifteen to thirty minutes in the tub nightly is still the norm, but the new tubs have all sorts of additional features—heating units, vibrators, bubble producers, earphones for music. In the opinion of this author, the Japanese are probably the most sophisticated bathers in the world, a tradition and custom that America is only beginning to emulate.

America

America has very little to contribute to bathing from a historical standpoint. However, as an interesting point, 1968 saw a new development—the invention of a whirlpool bath, known as the Jacuzzi. This was a whirlpool bath developed by a man named Roy Jacuzzi and shown first at a county fair as a therapeutic item for underwater massage, a concept that rapidly expanded into the whirlpool and hot tub rage that started in California in the 1970s and then expanded throughout the United States. To this day, people erroneously call any sort of whirlpool tub a Jacuzzi when, in fact, it was only one type of whirlpool bath. As you will see in a moment, the Jacuzzi is quite limited in scope in comparison to the hydrotherapy tubs that have come to us from Europe.

. . . .

SPA POINT

The important point to keep in mind with regard to history is simply that bathing is so important and has been a vital part of human life practically since the beginning of time. Nearly every culture in the world values bathing from a cleanliness, purification, religious, or well-being standpoint. More than four thousand years of bathing lead us to the day spa of today, perhaps the pinnacle of bathing practice.

. . . .

TERMINOLOGY

In order to establish the basis for bathing, it's important to understand some of the various terms used in relation to baths and bathing.

Hydrotherapy is the use of water in professional treatments for beautification and well-being. Hydrotherapy includes any and all modalities using water for treatment. This term is a generalized one for referring to water-based equipment and concepts.

Balneotherapy is the use of baths for beauty and therapeutic purposes. Using any bath constitutes use of this term.

Thalassotherapy is the use of seawater or seaweed for beautification and therapeutic purposes. It uses the mineral salts to help skin cells take up more oxygen, draw toxins out of the body, and feed the body naturally occurring minerals. Seawater is very close to blood plasma in composition, which may be partially why some of these benefits occur. The term, said to be coined in 1869 by the French doctor LaBonardiere d'Arcachon, was originally used for medical usages of seaweed and seawater. **Algotherapy** is another term for the use of algae, the official name for seaweed and sea grasses, in therapeutic treatments. Thalassotherapy is the more common term, hence recommended for the purposes of this book.

Herbal bath is the insertion of natural herbs or essences in baths for therapeutic effects. **Aromatherapy bath** would be another appropriate term. The technical difference between the two would depend on whether raw herbs or essential oils are used, aromatherapy being appropriate for the latter.

Whirlpool bath* is a type of bath in which air or water jets cause a bubbling or "whirling" effect in the water. There are whirlpool baths for professional use as well as personal home use and there are also attachments that can be added to a regular bathtub to cause a whirlpool tub effect. Normally multiple numbers of people can sit in the tub at one time. A **Jacuzzi bath*** is a whirlpool tub manufactured by the Jacuzzi company and sold by the name Jacuzzi. Usually this tub is large enough for multiple users at one time.

Hot tub* is normally a tub used privately in homes or "tub clubs," that may or may not be a whirlpool tub. The tub contains a heating element to

* These are not recommended for day spas for two primary reasons: from a multiple person usage, which can have a less than professional connotation, and from a hygienic standpoint. For sanitary reasons, the tub must be cleaned and sanitized properly between clients and this cannot be done in a cost or time effective manner.

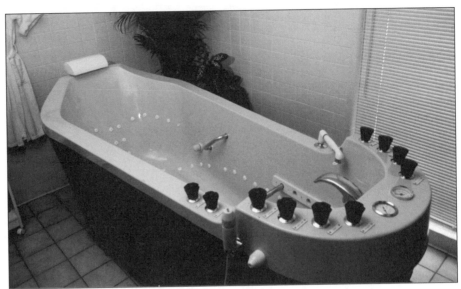

FIGURE 3-1 *Hydrotherapy tubs are designed with multiple air and water jets that can be operated at different pressures.*

keep the water warm. Hot tubs gained popularity in the late 1970s and 1980s and carry a connotation of partying and relaxation for fun. Hot tubs normally hold multiple persons.

Hydrotherapy tub is the ultimate in water treatment devices and the primary device discussed in this chapter. This is a tub specifically designed with multiple air and water jets for personal use (one person at a time only) and customized bath therapies (Figure 3-1). The tub, depending on the manufacturer, may have between 30 and 150 or so jets for air or water, strategically located in the tub and often pressure controlled in groups for different therapeutic purposes. Hydrotherapy tubs most often have an additional device, called the underwater massage hose, and attachments for underwater massage. The versatility of the hydrotherapy tub makes it a superior day spa piece of equipment. These tubs are quite expensive and require a wet room. They may not be appropriate for the beginner or a small operation. See the showers in the next chapter for alternatives.

Normal bath can be used for all the aspects of water treatment although a regular bathtub is not normally recommended for professional use. Tub treatments for home use will be discussed later, but even a plain tub can have whirlpool additions or bath additives, making it another viable form of hydrotherapy.

. . . .

SPA POINT

Whether offering plain water treatment or a herbal bath or a thalassotherapy treatment, the ultimate device for use is the hydrotherapy tub. This provides a very effective, versatile treatment capability for the individual client taking the treatment. Keep in mind the expense and space requirements.

. . . .

WHO TAKES THE BATHS?

As we know from history, bathing or taking tub baths has been a custom of people from all over the world. Although in modern America men traditionally take showers and women take baths, in reality emperors, kings, physicians, and even politicians have taken baths. It has been said that Winston Churchill took two baths a day to relax and clear his mind. Bathing in a tub, therefore, should not be considered a treatment only for women. A hydrotherapy tub treatment is viable for everyone—men, women, and children. It is interesting to consider that in a 1986 *Psychology Today* article, some of the family stress was attributed to the lack of enough bathrooms in the home. In house building today, the bathroom has become an important part of the "selling" of the house and often there are more bathrooms than bedrooms.

Hydrotherapy baths are recommended for medical purposes as well as for health maintenance. In the day spa, hydrotherapy baths with or without additives should be a big part of the overall well-being concept, and the wise day spa owner will further the effects of the hydrotherapy tub treatment by recommending baths at home as a follow-up, much in the same way as selling certain products for use at home following a facial treatment in the salon. Consistent bathing at home will more effectively enhance the results of the spa treatment.

WHAT HYDROTHERAPY TUB TREATMENTS DO

As will be reviewed often, water itself has a number of positive effects on the body, particularly in tub treatments. Water…

> … relaxes the body.
>
> … invigorates the body.
>
> … improves strength.
>
> … strengthens the immune system.
>
> … equalizes circulation and increases metabolism.
>
> … improves digestion and elimination.
>
> … enhances the penetration of other nutritional substances (additives in water).
>
> … relieves stiffness, soreness, and pain.
>
> … increases muscle tone and nerve functioning.

Warm to hot water lowers the blood pressure and pulls blood into the extremities, slowing blood as it is redistributed back to the heart, lungs, and central circulatory system. This is great for relaxation but may cause light-headedness. This can be dangerous for a client with a heart condition.

Through the improvement of circulation and elimination, we say that it has a detoxifying capability; it actually enhances the body's own detoxification process. Thus it also has a calming and sedative effect on the overall system and promotes homeostasis (the balance and harmony of all systems in the body).

NOTE: *Please review chapter 2 for further effects of hot and cold water.*

Who Should Not Take Hydrotherapy Baths— Contraindications

Persons with the following conditions should not receive hydrotherapy baths. Physician's release and instruction should be required.

*   High or low blood pressure or heart problems of any kind.

*   Pregnancy .

*   Significant obesity.

*   Systemic or chronic disease of any kind, especially cancer, AIDS, hepatitis, diabetes, seizures, hypo- or hyperthyroidism. Do only under physician recommendation and supervision.

*   Any infection or inflammatory condition.

*   Vascular problems such as phlebitis, varicose veins, or diabetes.

    Also keep in mind the following:

*   Do not offer treatment to any person under the influence of alcohol or drugs.

*   Do not do treatment to persons immediately after they have eaten a meal, particularly a big meal. Wait thirty minutes to an hour.

*   Although hydrotherapy is great for physical injuries such as tendonitis and sprains, be cautious and remember the effect of the lowering blood pressure over 95 degrees F.

*   Water agitated by jets can cause rashes or skin infections to spread. Do not do in cases of rashes or infections.

*   Do not allow your client to have very active exercise and then jump into a tub. Have client cool down prior to entering tub.

*   Avoid prolonged time in tub, particularly if not accustomed to it. Work time up from 5 minutes to 15 minutes to 20 or 30 minutes. Persons 65 years or older should be limited to 5–10 minutes at a time.

*   Treatment should be discontinued and client removed from tub in any and all cases of light-headedness, nausea, dizziness, heart palpitations, chest discomfort, headache, if having hot and cold chills, and in any other questionable condition.

*   Depending on the treatment, the client should not shave or wax any area for two days prior to treatment.

. . . .

SPA POINT

Although the contraindications mentioned may sound daunting and frightening at first, they are really just normal common sense issues, most of which are applicable even for a facial treatment. The difference and importance in caution lies in the fact that you are now treating the whole person and water therapy is quite active. The benefits and pleasures of hydrotherapy far outweigh the inconvenience of the contraindications. They must, however, not be ignored or forgotten.

. . . .

Rules of the Tub

1. There is no other more important situation in day spa treatments than in hydrotherapy and particularly tub-related treatments to have a good client health history. Before the client even has any type of body treatment, but particularly when hydrotherapy is involved, this history is imperative to protect the client as well as the technician and day spa. There is very little cause for concern overall, but it is important to know the contraindications mentioned previously and proceed carefully, especially when the client is new to hydrotherapy.

2. The client should not have a hydrotherapy tub treatment immediately after eating or strenuous exercise. Wait 30 minutes to 1 hour after eating and 15–20 minutes after strenuous exercise. You must not do any hydrotherapy treatments on clients after they have consumed alcohol.

3. It is also important that when the client is about to have a hydrotherapy tub treatment that he or she be reminded to use the restroom before treatment. It is very common to have to stop a treatment midcourse to allow the client to use the facilities anyway, but it is always a good idea to go before.

4. The client should undress and if possible take a quick warm shower before entering the tub room. If a shower is not possible, be sure the client is comfortably robed after undressing. You do not want the client to get a chill.

5. If the client has never had any type of treatment, whether to wear a bathing suit or not should be discussed. It is much better and more effective to do any and all body treatments and hydrotherapy treatments with the client nude. The client must feel comfortable, and draping, robing, and averting eyes at specific times is important.

6. After all hydrotherapy treatment, the client should be given water (flavored waters are good) or juice to help replenish the potassium lost in treatment. Orange juice is probably the best.

7. During the hydrotherapy tub treatment, a cool cloth can be applied to the client's head. Do not use ice cold cloths as they may cause a headache. If the client becomes thirsty offer cool, not cold, water.

8. Under no circumstance is the client to be left entirely alone during a tub treatment. He/she can overrelax, fall asleep, faint, and drown! If you leave the room, do so only momentarily and then stand by.

9. This will be discussed more fully in *Day Spa Operations*, but it's vital to purchase a tub with a power draining system, to have good enough drainage in your plumbing system to have the tub drain very quickly, and to have a hot water heater adequate for your needs. Many day spas have only 60-gallon tanks, which is often not enough. Consider 100-gallon tanks.

NOTE: *The specifics of client preparation, room setup, etc. will be discussed in the applicable chapters, mostly in chapter 7. You should also refer to* Day Spa Operations, *the companion business book, for more information.*

Tub Temperatures

Although, as previously discussed, cool and cold water are invigorating and highly recommended for treatment, the practical reality in day spas today in America is that the typical client is very averse to cold treatment at all. It's quite common in spas in Europe to combine hot and cold therapy as a matter of course, but when the same concept is done on the inexperienced spa goer in this country, you will find great resistance and often a very dissatisfied client. Cold water therapy should be offered with caution and only to the experienced spa client and should be discussed in advance. So in simple terms, keep the water warm!

WATER TEMPERATURES IN DEGREES F	
Cold Bath:	50–70
Cool Bath:	70–80
Tepid Bath:	80–94
Warm Bath:	94–98
Hot Bath:	98–105

Extremely hot baths for the very healthy and experienced person may go as high as 115–120 degrees F, but is not normally recommended because anything over 105 degrees can cause the blood pressure to plummet and seriously stress the heart (at 95 degrees the blood pressure begins to drop). An ideal range would normally be in the mid-90s (between 93 and 95) with nothing over 100 degrees for the inexperienced.

Your tub may register the temperature on a meter or you may wish to have a water thermometer (Figure 3-2). Another method of checking the client would be to use a pulse rate measurement on the client. Some tubs come with a pulse rate meter where the client can have a band attached to the finger. The maximum pulse rate suggested would be no more than 120. This method isn't always accurate. Therefore, it is important to stay with the client during tub treatments and be sure the client is comfortable and is

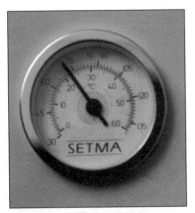

FIGURE 3-2 *Water temperatures in hydrotherapy tubs are controlled by meters.*

not getting overheated or light-headed or developing a headache. In any case where this might happen, the treatment needs to be discontinued. Also remember that if the tub has air or water jets, as the water is circulated the temperature will increase, so watch the temperature during treatment and add cold water to the tub as necessary to maintain a comfortable mid-90 degrees.

SUMMARY OF TUB TEMPERATURE
- Average temperature should be kept at mid-90 degrees, around 93–95.

- Never go over 105 degrees.

- Temperature increases with air and water flow in tub. Watch meter and keep temperature down.

- Lower temperatures are better for the inexperienced.

- Light-headedness is a strong sign to discontinue treatment.

. . . .

SPA POINT
Although many people think they want a very hot bath, temperatures over 105 degrees F can cause a serious drop in blood pressure and stress on the heart. Ideal temperatures for a bath should be around the mid-90s for safety and relaxation.

. . . .

Treatment Times

The length of treatment time in a tub varies according to a number of issues, the main one being the goal of the treatment. If the treatment is simple with little or no additives tub time in a tepid to warm tub can be up to 30 minutes. If, however, the tub is hot, additives are highly active, underwater massage is going to be performed, or other treatments will follow, time in the tub should be drastically reduced. Although treatments are offered only to healthy persons, even the novice healthy person can easily become light-headed; thus treatment times should start low and be increased according to the client's comfort level. Initially, most treatments are safe for 15 minutes, gradually increasing to 30 minutes maximum.

For textbook normalization, the rest time after tub time should be equal. That is to say, if the person is in the tub for 30 minutes, then rest time should also be 30 minutes. In the day spa environment, this is difficult, if not impractical to expect. Therefore, rest time combined with consultation or booking another service afterwards is the safest answer to client balancing. Beginners and persons over 60 years of age with normal health histories should start between 5–15 minutes. Highly healthy, active, well-exercised individuals may begin with 15–20 minutes working up to 30 minutes within three treatments. In most situations baths could be done daily, but it's more realistic to assume a client will take a bath once in a while if just for relaxation. If the goal is for slimming or anticellulite, then a frequency of 2–3 times a week is much more effective.

```
TUB TIME

First to third times:              5–15 minutes
Inexperienced, over 60 years old:  5–15 minutes
Generally healthy/active:          15–25 minutes
Experienced:                       20–30 minutes
```

ALTERNATING BATHS

Generally speaking, warm baths are relaxing, cold baths are stimulating. Alternating warm and cold baths are a great form of therapy but the time for the cold bath should be much less than the warm bath. As a safe example, 1 minute of very cold to 5 minutes of warm or 2 minutes of cool to 6 minutes of warm is ideal to maintain the stimulus without letting the cold faction depress bodily functions. Be very cautious about going back and forth between warm and cold baths, especially when the temperature differential is great.

. . . .

SPA POINT

Alternating warm and cold is probably the ideal situation but not practical most of the time in America for the inexperienced spa goer. Temperature is critically important to achieve the results of the treatments without depressing or enervating the body. From a safety standpoint, lower warm temperatures are always safer.

. . . .

AIR AND WATER JETS

Each manufacturer should educate you specifically on the proper use of that tub. There are many variations in options and the best instructor will be the manufacturer. Keep the following in mind.

- In some tubs, the addition of air and water jets quickly increases the water temperature. Watch the temperature gauge carefully.

- All jets should be well covered with water before being turned on to avoid sudden splashes of water out of the tub or taking the chance of ruining the motor.

- Client should enter the tub without any jets on at all. If applicable, the jets should then be pointed to the specific areas planned for concentration.

- Before turning on the jets, the client should be informed on what to expect and which jets are coming on. Then normally air jets are turned on first to cause an overall bubbling, invigorating sensation. Be sure the client is holding on to the handles for balance and support. Most tubs also have foot bars to help keep the client in position. Be sure all positions are explained prior to turning jets on.

- Water jets are then strategically turned on according to a plan if the tub has this capability. In most cases, water jets are started working from the feet to the back of the neck. Jets then run for the specified amount of time. Normally the time in a 30-minute treatment is about 10 minutes. Then additives or underwater massage is the next step. Then once again the client relaxes with the jets bubbling for the last 10 minutes.

NOTE: *Refer to manufacturers for specific training on their product.*

WARM UP:	10 minutes, jets alone
TREATMENT:	10 minutes, bath additives and/or underwater massage
COOL DOWN:	10 minutes, add cool water and tone down.
For the inexperienced client, cut time in half.	

· ·

SPA POINT

The highlight of having a professional hydrotherapy tub is the wonderful features of air and water jets and all the combinations of treatment that can be accomplished. Do not, however, overdo the treatment, and remember that the jets cause the water temperature to increase. The turbulence of the water can also be very enervating to the client, so close watch over the client is imperative.

· ·

UNDERWATER MASSAGE

The hose and attachments vary from one tub to the next. The overall goal of hose usage is to perform underwater massage (Figure 3-3). Although a client could possibly manipulate the hose by him- or herself, this is never recommended. This is strictly a professional treatment for the knowledgeable technician. Underwater massage can be used for the following purposes.

1. Underwater massage provides water resistance for passive muscle exercise to strengthen weak muscles or tone up muscles, increase or restore joint motion, clean and stimulate the healing of burned flesh, and aid in muscle function. (Avoid these medical uses.)

2. Underwater massage is a very effective stimulant for the breakup and dissolution of cellulite. Multiple treatments are required.

3. Underwater massage will increase circulation and stimulate skin function.

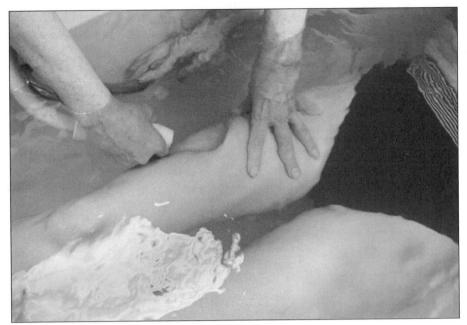

FIGURE 3-3 *An underwater hose can direct pressure at specific parts of the body for targeted massage.*

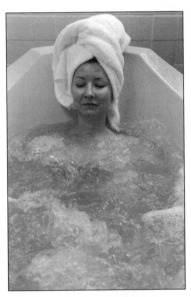

FIGURE 3-4 *Clients can relax in a hydrotherapy bath as the water swirls over and massages their entire body.*

Use of the Hose

4. Providing the technician has been trained in manual lymph drainage, the hose may be used for a mechanical underwater manual lymph drainage massage, often called *aqua drainage.*

5. Underwater massage feels very relaxing and invigorating to the client.

6. The swirling of water over the legs, arms, and back provides the entire person with a sense of well-being (Figure 3-4).

Depending on the goal of treatment, specific hose training should be provided by the manufacturer.

Be sure the hose is placed well into the lower part of the water before it is turned on and be sure to have a good hold on it. If the hose escapes the technician's hand while on, it may fly and splash everywhere, not to mention the danger of hitting and injuring the client. Throughout the treatment, the hose must be kept underwater. Also always keep the nozzle pointed in the direction of flow, toward the heart. Keep fingers of the hand holding the nozzle over it to gauge pressure. The pressure from the hose should be at a comfortable level for the client. (The manufacturer should make specific recommendations.)

The underwater massage normally begins at the bottom of the foot and slowly proceeds with smooth, comfortable, circular movements. Generally speaking all movements work toward the heart (Figure 3-5). The amount of time for the underwater massage should be between 5 and 10 minutes, no more than 15 minutes. This is very active exercise and can easily tire the client.

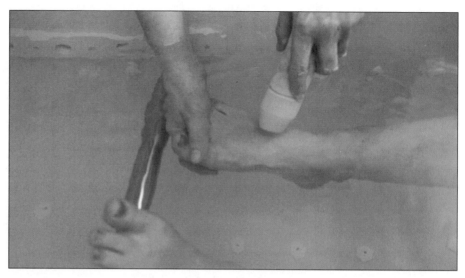

FIGURE 3-5 An underwater hose directs pressure at the foot.

NOTE: Be sure to advise the client that underwater massage will most often cause the client to have to use the restroom immediately after treatment and often for several hours after.

PROCEDURE

1. Starting from the base of the foot circle the soles up and over to the top of the foot, up the inside of the leg to the groin, then again up the outside of the leg to the buttocks. When doing the outside of the leg, circle the knee a few times. Pressure should never be applied directly on lymph nodes (behind the knees, groin, axilla, base of neck at clavicle, etc.)

2. Moving now from the top of the leg, continue to circle up the sides of the legs. Then have the client turn to the side slightly in order to do the buttocks and work up that side of the back (Figure 3-6). The back should be done in sections beginning with smooth movements up the center of the spine and down to the base of the back, out to the sides and in rows from the spine out to the sides working up to the shoulders.

NOTE: If the client is having a cellulite problem or a cellulite treatment is to follow, extra time should be spent on areas of the cellulite. Depending on the situation, pressure may be increased for this area.

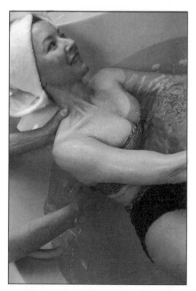

FIGURE 3-6 The client turns slightly so that the water pressure from the hose can massage the back.

3. The client lies back and the shoulders and neck are done while the client lies low in the water. The client's neck must be below the surface of the water for the hose to be effective without splashing. The back and neck are normally worked more than other parts due to typical stress and tension in those areas.

4. The hose is then taken back to the other foot and the procedure is repeated for the other leg and that side of the body.

5. If the abdominal area is to be done, great care must be taken. It is normally the last area to be done, and the pressure should be lowered. The movement for the stomach should be in a clockwise direction beginning at the lower left-hand side of the stomach and moving gently and slowly in a square following the flow of the colon around the navel. When the right lower corner is reached, the hose is lifted and replaced at the starting point. Do not make a full circle. This causes backward movement in the lower middle quadrant and can be very uncomfortable for the client.

Underwater Massage Contraindications

In addition to the contraindications for tub treatments in general, the activity of the underwater massage greatly stimulates the system. Therefore, this should not be done in any questionable health issue, on anemic or systemically weak persons, chronic systemic diseases, vascular problems (varicose veins, phlebitis, hemophilia, diabetes). Watch the client's blood pressure or comfort level at all times, and should light-headedness or overheating occur stop treatment.

TUB TREATMENTS

In general there are three major categories of tub treatments available:

1. Plain water baths—no additives, with or without underwater massage.

2. Thalassotherapy baths—additives of seaweed, seawater, sea salts, and sometimes sea mud.

3. Aromatherapy or herbal baths—additives of herbs or essential oils.

As you have already learned, even a plain bath has tremendous effects. However, the addition of seaweed or aromatherapy essences can tremendously enhance the bath. The combination of seaweed, salts, and essential oils is also very common. The decision of what to put in the baths is a matter of personal preference, experience, or manufacturer recommendations. There can be hundreds of combinations. Depending on the number of essential oils you carry, the combinations can be endless. Seaweed, seawater, and sea salts vary in composition according to the supplier as well so choose the sea-based product according to the manufacturer's recommendation.

The additives should be put in after the client has relaxed in the tub for 5 to 10 minutes unless otherwise specified by the manufacturer. Proper amounts should also be designated by the manufacturer, so the suggestions that follow will not specify amounts. Keep in mind that there may also be other additives such as mud or milk, but these are less common.

As an aside, for those who are intrigued by Kneipp baths and concepts, his overall concept was based on the idea of alternating cold and warm baths. For various baths, he used hay flower to open pores and to dissolve toxins. This was his all-purpose bath. He also used oat straw for kidney and elimination problems and pine sprigs for strengthening the blood vessels and for aged people. He had numerous combinations. Today the Kneipp Corporation offers a number of different bath combinations and products.

Thalassotherapy

> CAUTION: IF THE CLIENT HAS ANY ALLERGIES TO IODINE, SEAWEED MUST NOT BE USED!

Seaweed baths increase metabolism and blood circulation, activate the exchanges of substances in the body, and increase the elimination of toxins and waste materials. Seaweed is high in Vitamins A, B_1, B_2, B_{12}, C, D, E, and K and helps re-energize the whole body. The mineral salts act on cell vitality, help in skin moisturization, and assist in smoothing and retexturizing the skin. The iodine in seaweed can facilitate the slimming process and works like thyroid to help activate metabolism, circulation, and revitalization of cells. Seaweed in baths also facilitates the relaxation of muscles (Figure 3-7).

> NOTE: *See chapter 11 for more detailed information on seaweeds and the various species as there are more than 25,000 different types.*

RELAXING BATH

Blue-green:	*Spirulina*
Brown:	*Fucus, Ascophyllum nodosum*
Red:	*Chondrus, Corallina*

Spirulina is rich in vitamins and beta carotene and is effective to reduce fatigue and stimulate metabolism.

Fucus and *Ascophyllum nodosum* are rich in vitamins and amino acids to relax and to neutralize free radicals.

Chondrus and *Corallina* are both remineralizers and revitalizers.

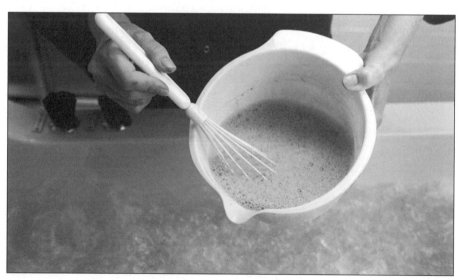

FIGURE 3-7 *Mix dry seaweed and water and pour into the bath.*

```
┌─────────────────────────────────────────────┐
│ INVIGORATING BATH                             │
│                                               │
│ Blue:    Spirulina                            │
│ Brown:   Laminaria, Fucus, Macrocystis        │
│ Green:   Chlorella                            │
└─────────────────────────────────────────────┘
```

Laminaria is rich in minerals and amino acids to increase metabolism and may stimulate thyroid activity.

Fucus and Macrocystis have high iodine content to also stimulate metabolism, and the high potassium content remineralizes the body and plays an important role in cellular transport.

Chlorella contains iron, vitamin B$_3$, chlorophyl, and nucleic acids. It is used for its regenerating effect and stimulation of circulation.

These seaweeds may be chosen alone or combined as desired. Most manufacturers will have already combined various seaweeds for your use. Normally one bath utilizes 4–6 ounces of seaweed in powder form. Powders should be mixed with warm water in a bowl and then added to the bath. If underwater massage is also to be performed, reduce the amount of seaweed so as to be able to see through the water.

Aromatherapy Baths

As you will learn in chapter 6, the hundreds of essences available can make treatment very complicated. However, it's best to start with just a few and learn as you go. Although you may wish to add four or more essential oils, it may be a better idea to use only three initially until you have a good understanding of the effects of aromatherapy. Some essential oils can counteract others. Additionally, since these are aromatic essences, each technician has her own favorite combinations.

The following combinations include more than three oils in some cases, so please combine three of your choice. The general acceptable amounts of oils for baths would be 10–30 drops if the essential oil is in a carrier oil and no more than 10 drops of pure essences (Figure 3-8). Do not exceed this amount unless your manufacturer specifically suggests otherwise. The following combinations are only suggestions. You may also wish to follow the chart and information from chapter 6 for other combinations. Also, refer to your manufacturers for specific recommendations.

RELAXING:	lavender, clary sage, melissa, ylang ylang, bergamot, chamomile
STIMULATING:	rosemary, thyme, lavender (good for toning), pine, cypress
SOOTHING:	chamomile, jasmine, geranium, rose
MOISTURIZING:	orange blossom, neroli, patchouli, lavender
CONTOURING:	pine, thyme, camphor, juniper

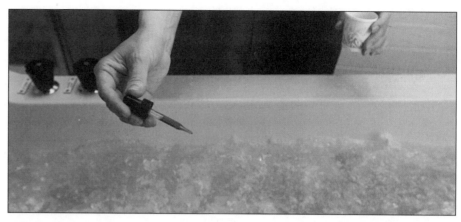

FIGURE 3-8 *Drops of essential oils in water provide an aromatherapy treatment along with the benefits of underwater massage.*

Keep in mind that most bathing concepts are based on three issues: relaxation, stimulation and invigoration, and anticellulite treatment.

. . . .

SPA POINT

There is nothing more wonderful and invigorating than a thalassotherapy bath, particularly with essential oils. The treatment heightens the effects of the tub and water dramatically. Various combinations of essential oils and seaweeds can be offered and the client will never become bored.

. . . .

Hydrotherapy Tub Treatment

PROCEDURE

1. Client undresses and showers.

2. The client is escorted to the tub room, and the procedure to take place is explained. Contraindications, medications, and so forth should be reiterated even if this is a repeat client.

3. The client sits on the edge of the tub, swings legs over, and enters the tub with the help of the technician. The tub has already been filled with water, but normally the additives haven't been put in yet.

4. The technician helps get the client comfortably seated with head resting on the pillow and feet on the footrest or under the foot protective bar. Client's hands should be placed on the handrails. Once the client is comfortable, the treatment begins.

5. Turn on air and water jets according to the manufacturer's directions. While the client relaxes for the first 10 minutes, additives are mixed and added to the tub. This is a good time to discuss seaweed, mud, aromatherapy, or whatever additive has been put in the tub.

6. The underwater massage is then performed with the hose if applicable to the treatment.

7. Sometimes at this point the water is cooled down a little for the last 10 minutes of the treatment. This will depend on the treatment, condition of the client, and so forth. The client's comfort and how he/she feels should be inquired about periodically during the 30-minute treatment.

End of the Bath Treatment

As stated already, if the client isn't having another treatment, the ideal situation is to rest for a time equal to the treatment time. This isn't practical in most day spas so the ideal situation is to have the client receive some treatment after the bath—manicure or hairstyle or a full-body massage. If the client only has a bath, try to use the resting time to educate the client on home care procedures and products.

PROCEDURE

1. When the bath is completed after the cool down time, the water and air jets should all be stopped.

2. The client stands and sits on the edge of the tub facing the inside of the tub.

3. Slowly the client swings legs over the edge with the technician's help. Be sure to have a towel on the floor so that the client doesn't slip.

4. The technician wraps the client in a robe. Do not bother drying the client with towels. The robe should be put on over the wet body.

5. The client is then escorted to the rest area or restroom. Then the client is given a small glass of juice or water to sip slowly. Juice is good. The client is then consulted with and products are discussed. If another treatment is to be done, this process will be done at the end of all treatments.

CLEANING THE TUB AND ROOM

Although this will be covered also in another chapter, it must be stressed that hydrotherapy tub treatments are only as good as the sanitation and hygienic practices in the spa. The tub must be cleaned and disinfected between each client. This doesn't just mean to drain the tub and wipe it out. Remember, there are jets in the tub and these must also be cleaned out and then the whole tub rinsed and dried. The room should also be sanitized and wiped down with a towel. The floors should be sanitized and dried. This is a must for a successful operation. If this is not done, clients will soon discontinue having treatments and may even begin talking badly about the general hygiene in the spa. If you want a hydrotherapy tub and intend to make it successful, the cleaning importance cannot be stressed enough and employees must know this well at the outset.

Synopsis

Hydrotherapy is the pinnacle of day spa treatments. The hydrotherapy tub may be expensive but it will also offer a versatility and sophistication of treatment no other modality will offer. The physiological benefits of hydrotherapy are in relaxation, metabolic improvement, relief of fatigue, detoxification, skin conditioning, and stress relief. There are also cautions that must be kept in mind. But the most exciting aspect of hydrotherapy lies in the ability to grow and continue learning and to help the client on an ongoing basis for many many years. The psychological benefits are too numerous to mention, not only for the client but also for the technician. It's a wonderful therapy with history, efficacy, and great pleasure.

Review

1. How do we know that the Romans were famous for bathing?
2. Who was Roy Jacuzzi?
3. What is the difference between balneotherapy and thalassotherapy?
4. What makes a hydrotherapy tub special?
5. List three contraindications to hydrotherapy bath treatments.
6. What is the ideal temperature range for tub treatments?
7. What does underwater massage do for the client?
8. What are the three major categories of tub treatments?
9. Name two seaweeds recommended for use in tub treatments.
10. Name three essential oils used for relaxation baths.

CHAPTER 4
Showers _____

OVERVIEW

Showers of some form or another have existed since the beginning of water usage. From the simplest form of pouring a cup of water over the head to the sophisticated showers we have today, showers present another form of hydrotherapy. Whether you realize it or not, every morning or evening when you are taking your shower you're actually having a hydrotherapy treatment. In fact, as we have discussed in chapter 2 on what water does for the human organism, a shower format for application of water greatly enhances water therapy. Many salons that don't want to add a shower but want to call themselves day spas are missing the quick and effective benefits of a shower. The plain shower you have in your home is, in actuality, a form of hydrotherapy if you think of it that way and utilize it for its fullest value. A salon desiring to convert to a day spa concept must, at the very least, add a shower. The problem is that nobody gives much thought to the shower since everyone has one at home, but there can be much more to the shower than you think.

Then there are also the more sophisticated variations to the shower—the Vichy shower, the steam shower, the Swiss shower, and others. Each of these showers have similar functions and variations. The day spa may choose to add one or all to the spa system according to needs and space requirements. The beauty of having several variations of showers lies in the versatility and ability to do different treatments with each. So, let's look at how each one may be used in the day spa.

. . . .

SPA POINT

It's amazing to consider the fact that a regular shower, similar to what everyone has in their home, is actually a vital hydrotherapy device if used as such. The shower is a basic requirement of a proper day spa.

. . . .

THE REGULAR SHOWER

As stated, a regular shower is a must for a salon to convert to a day spa in the opinion of this author. The shower is used for a number of purposes. When the client takes a quick shower prior to a body treatment, the purpose of this is threefold.

1. To be sure that the client is clean. The client must use soap and really cleanse.

2. Normally the initial shower will be a warm shower to prepare the client for treatment by warming and relaxing muscles and tension. This warming has an important effect on the body and helps whatever treatment is taking place after that work better.

3. It not only gives the technician the impression that the client is clean, but also buys time to make the treatment area ready and customized for this specific client.

The shower will be used to rinse off products from treatments, such as seaweed, mud, and exfoliants. If a shower is the only water modality, its importance will increase. The shower can be a place for hot or cold showers, or alternating hot and cold depending on the goal, short or long showers depending on the treatment, or a combination. If the shower is actually to be used as a specific treatment modality, it's wise to get a shower head system that allows for various water selections and pressures. The shower head or hand-held hose will convert a simple shower to a water massage device as well. The hand-held shower may also be used for local treatment, for example, in a situation where there may be a sore joint or swelling you may want the client to cold shower just that area for several minutes.

Rules of the Shower

The shower must be cleaned, disinfected, and dried between clients. This includes the shower, shower curtain, and floor outside the shower. Absolute perfect sanitary practices will preserve your business. It's not an extra, it's law so be sure that you inform new staff during the interview and be sure it's in the job description. They soon tire of this mundane job and then you have a problem, unless you hire a person specifically for cleaning purposes. This is not cost effective in a very small salon but is quite worthwhile in a large salon. It's better use of your employees to have your technicians working and selling from one client to the next rather than losing a product sale because they need to clean the shower.

The only products allowed in the shower should be soaps, shower gels, and shampoos that you sell. Do not put a bar of soap in the shower for multiple person usage. If you insist on bar soap, be sure it's the amenity size (like the soaps you receive at a hotel). The shower is not only a place for the client to get clean and receive professional treatment, it's actually one of your best retail centers in the entire day spa. It will, of course, cost you some money because the client will use your product, but that's exactly what you want. Be sure the shower has your liquid soaps, sponges, or shammy, and whatever else you want that client to use. The dispensers you find in health clubs are fine only if they are well labelled with your product. The typical consumer thought about dispenser product is cheap. If you give that impression, you're in trouble. It's actually more impressive to use retail size containers and refill them (yes, it's a hassle, but the sales will prove it worthwhile to you in short order).

Every time the client gets out of the shower, there should be a fresh new clean bath towel. Do not make the client reuse the same towel two or three times. This is unprofessional and also gives a cheap impression. The bath mat should also be changed after each client. In a spa situation, a towel may be better and less expensive.

Don't allow the client to be in the shower longer than you specifically direct. Some consumers will stand in the shower for days before you can get them out and this will throw you behind. You should stay with the client and make conversation or do something to keep them moving right along. This rule will be true of all showers. Also, don't let the client take a shower that is too hot. Remember, very hot water will lower blood pressure and if the client fainted in the shower, you could have problems. Always remain with the client while going to the shower and remain nearby while client is in the shower. This is for safety as well as to move the client along.

SHOWER TREATMENTS
Regular Shower

WARM-UPS AND RINSES
Always have the client shower initially and shampoo the body to get clean. Then the rinse time should be about 3 minutes to rinse well and also to relax. Later, when the shower is being used to rinse a product off, the rinse should be about 5 minutes long. If the client has become chilled from moving from the treatment area to the shower, allow enough time in the shower for warming the body again.

THE COLD SHOWER
A cold shower, as we discussed in previous chapters, is very invigorating. A cool to cold shower can be used to invigorate the body and contract the skin. The cold shower would normally be taken after the warm shower or treatment as a finisher to rev up the system. If the client is in the warm shower for 5-6 minutes, the amount of time in the cold shower would be about 1-2 minutes. This is quite sufficient. If you have a hand-held nozzle, the cold shower can be directed at areas of swelling or soreness to comfort those areas. Keep in mind you are not specifically medically treating the area. The cold shower can also be alternated with warm. In a regular shower this is a bit difficult sometimes depending on the water heating/cooling time. Other showers are more effective for this but if this is all you have, it will work anyway. Maximum time for alternating hot and cold would be 12-15 minutes, with the cold time being about one-third of the warm time.

RINSING
Using the shower for rinsing may take place as many as three times or more during a treatment depending on all the steps to the treatment, so it's important to make sure that the rinsing is done quickly. Of course the first shower is the cleansing shower when the client first arrives, and soap or shower gel should be used. Thereafter, unless specified by the technician, rinsing is done without soaping up again. The rinse should normally be warm and done within 1 minute or so. While the client is rinsing, the technician will be changing the bed, preparing for the next step, and so forth. However, the technician should always take the client to the shower and remain close by.

PRICE

Showers run $800 and up.

The Swiss Shower

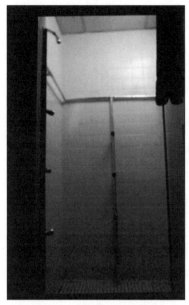

FIGURE 4-1 *The Swiss shower surrounds the bather with water. Streams of water can be concentrated to specific areas of the body.*

The Swiss shower is a wonderful addition to a normal shower cabinet or stall. As sophisticated as the name implies, the Swiss shower of today is far less complicated than it was twenty years ago. Just a few decades ago, the Swiss shower was often called the circular shower because the person would stand inside what looked somewhat like a coil. There were six to ten rows of steel surrounding the bather with hundreds of holes in the pipes for the water to come out (Figure 4-1). The goal of the shower was and is to concentrate a stream of water at common strategic areas.

Nowadays, this same thing is accomplished by having pipes in all four corners of the shower with eight to sixteen heads emanating from each corner. Again the regions concentrated on would be divided into thirds, with the upper row concentrated at the upper torso, middle row to the stomach/lower back region, and the lower row to the hips and thigh region. An important thing to keep in mind about the Swiss shower is the fact that since it's a therapeutic shower device, an overhead shower head is not normally part of the system. It is wise, however, to be sure the shower stall is plumbed for a regular overhead shower as well in order to have double duty with this tool. The best aspect of the Swiss shower is that it takes only as much room as is normally needed for a regular shower. The special treatment aspect of the Swiss shower is the hot and cold alternating treatment with pulsation capability. Normally, the client enters the shower, but the strength, temperature, and pressure is controlled by the technician from a control panel on the wall outside the shower. The client merely stands in the shower and the rest is handled from the technician's side.

Remember, as such the Swiss shower is for hydrotherapy, water treatment, and is therefore not really much used for a regular shower washing. The main goal is water pressure therapy in a mild way. This adds to the flair of the therapeutic treatment and to the marketability of the shower. It's really quite a nice shower and can easily be incorporated into packages with add-on charges and very little effort on the part of the technician.

• •

SPA POINT

The Swiss shower is a great asset because it can be included in a regular shower and adds tremendous dimension to the treatment capability. It also offers added benefits by being able to alternate hot and cold water treatment.

• •

RULES OF THE SWISS SHOWER

• Client should not use immediately after eating.

• Be sure the shower stall has handles on the wall for the client to hold onto.

• The shower temperature should alternate between warm and cold in the same ratio as mentioned earlier. Temperatures must be comfortable and adjusted to each client.

- Maximum time in the shower should be no more than 15 minutes. This should be adjusted down according to the tolerance of the client.

- The direction of the shower heads should be adjusted to the size of the client. There's nothing worse than having a short person in the shower being pummeled in the neck with water.

The Swiss shower is normally marketed in conjunction with some other service, not by itself. It can be, of course, but not normally.

SAMPLE TREATMENT

1. Client enters spa for treatment, undresses, and takes a normal cleansing shower.

2. The technician then adjusts the Swiss shower and operates the control panel with alternating warm/cool showering for 5 to 10 or 12 minutes. The controls and temperatures should be trained specifically by the manufacturer.

3. When the shower is completed, the client is removed, robed, and moved to a treatment room where any number of treatments can be performed. A simple combination would be the Swiss shower and 30-minute massage. This makes a good one-hour overall treatment. If the client merely wants the Swiss shower, apply a finishing lotion, discuss home care, and the treatment is complete. The application of the lotion will serve as the resting time that should follow the hydrotherapy shower treatment.

NOTE: *Normally products are not specified for the Swiss shower treatment phase itself but may be applied before or after according to the need. As an example, an anticellulite gel or cream may be applied prior to entering the shower and then the shower may facilitate the heating process.*

PRICE
Swiss showers normally run from $2,000 to $5,000.

The Vichy Shower

A favorite of this author, the Vichy shower offers great marketability and versatility to a wet room. As will be discussed in chapter 7, the wet room is just that, a room that can become wet. The wet room is normally tiled from floor to ceiling, well drained, with lighting and ventilation to accommodate steam and warming. In simple terms, the Vichy shower is a horizontal rod with holes to allow water raining or cascading from above the bed or table (Figure 4-2). The Vichy shower is situated about 4 feet above the bed, which can also become wet, where the client is lying. Some spas use tiled tables, but these are very uncomfortable. Some use special water foam pads over metal that doesn't rust or plastic tables.

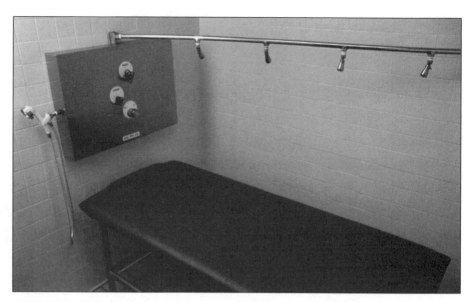

FIGURE 4-2 *The Vichy shower rains water onto the bather as he or she lies on the bed or table.*

The Vichy shower can be used as a rinsing device but it is really much more. It is designed to alternate and pulsate hot and cold water. The water pressure is such that the effect on the client is a comfortable raining effect. The water flow, temperature, and pulsation are controlled by the technician from a control panel. This panel is normally at the end of the bed where the pole emanates (Figure 4-3). The technician will often get somewhat wet, and should dress appropriately to do Vichy shower treatments. As with all shower treatments, once the controls are set and the treatment is taking place, the technician should stand close by, maybe not in the room to allow the client to relax, but immediately outside. It cannot be stressed often enough that the client is never left alone in hydrotherapy treatments. If the lighting is subdued, with soft music, the raining effect of the shower is wonderfully therapeutic and obviously goes well beyond just rinsing something off the body.

Although a client can book just the Vichy shower treatment alone, it is better to combine it with a salt glow, mud treatment, or seaweed wrap for a number of reasons, the primary one being the need to rinse these substances off anyway, but also to more cost effectively use the wet room. Salt glow, mud, and seaweed wraps are ideally done in a wet room to facilitate removal anyway. The addition of the Vichy shower greatly enhances the chargability of the service.

· ·

SPA POINT

The Vichy shower makes a wet room salt, mud, or seaweed treatment a wonderful experience as well as facilitating the removal of items with less effort on the part of the client or technician. The shower can be used multiple times during the treatment.

· ·

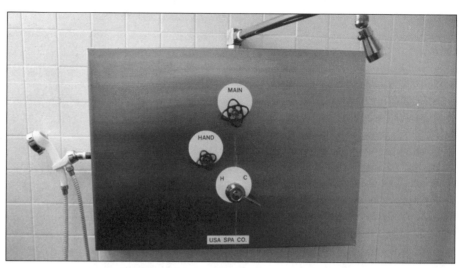

FIGURE 4-3 *The technician controls the shower with an operating panel, located at the end of the bed.*

RULES OF THE VICHY SHOWER

- Client should not use immediately after eating.

- When the client is about to be positioned on the table, be sure the Vichy shower pole doesn't hit the client in the head. If the pole is on a swivel, move the bar out of the way.

- The hand-held shower hose can be used to test water temperature.

- If your Vichy shower has a plastic face guard, be sure it is positioned well to protect the client's face as much as possible from the shower. Inevitably some water will reach the client's face, but try to keep it off the face as much as possible. If there is no guard, give the client a moist hand towel or skin shammy to put over the face.

- Technician must be prepared to get wet. Changes of clothes or water-proof clothes and shoes should be considered. Even if the control panel is mounted outside the Vichy shower, which is very expensive, working on the client in the wet area will still cause some water splashing and wet feet.

- When the client is asked to turn over, the technician should be right with the client assuring that he/she doesn't roll or slip off the table. The client is instructed to turn toward the technician and the technician holds the client's waist while turning. The turning of the client should be done slowly to prevent light-headedness or dizziness. This is particularly important if the client is lying in mud or seaweed that can be very slippery.

- Great care must be taken in getting the client up and off the table. The area may be slippery and the client will normally be quite relaxed so allow the client to sit up and stabilize for a couple of minutes before robing and leaving the room. A wet towel must be placed on the floor before the client gets out.

SAMPLE TREATMENT WITH VICHY SHOWER

1. Client enters spa, undresses, and takes normal cleansing shower. After robing, client is taken to the wet room. Some wet rooms also have a shower in the room, so the client may shower in the treatment room.

2. The technician then helps the client onto the table and instructs the client about what is going to take place while helping him/her lie down on stomach (if only the Vichy shower is being done, client will lie on back). The head should be placed at the end of the shower where the face shield is. The treatment product is then applied, for example, if doing a salt glow, the entire back side of the body is salted (see chapter 9), then the client rolls over and the front side is salted.

3. The Vichy shower is turned on and allowed to rain on the client for the appropriate amount of time depending on the treatment. If using just to remove the salt, 2–3 minutes will be sufficient. If the treatment is combined and the Vichy is a charged service, the time will normally be about 10 minutes.

4. The client is rolled over onto stomach again and the Vichy shower procedure is repeated. Be sure all residue of salt has been washed away. The hose on the Vichy shower will be used to rinse all final bits away. The shower phase is completed for the salt glow. If a mud or seaweed is to follow, the shower treatment will be repeated for the removal of the product but normally with less raining time. If both salt glow and seaweed or mud are done, the Vichy shower time should be divided equally out with a total Vichy shower time of 15–20 minutes at most. Both along with the Vichy shower can be done easily in 1 hour.

5. After the shower has been turned off, a finishing body lotion will be applied to the back side, the client rolls over onto the back, and the lotion is applied to the front side. If a dry room is available, it's much better to apply the lotion and massage it there. It is, however, a little more time consuming, and uses more towels.

6. The client is helped to a sitting position and allowed to stabilize for a few minutes before getting off the table. The client is escorted to the restroom, then to rest or next treatment area, given water or juice, and the next procedure begins or the client is consulted on products and treatments.

TREATMENT COMBINATIONS WITH VICHY SHOWER

Vichy Shower Treatment by Itself

Book 45 minutes. Client is on table for about 20 minutes. Finishing lotion is applied and treatment completed in 30 minutes, and 15 minutes is allowed for cleanup, changeover, sales.

Vichy Shower/Salt Glow

Book 1 hour. Client receives the salt exfoliation on front side in about 15 minutes, back side about 10 minutes, 10 minutes for the Vichy shower in total, 10 minutes for lotion application. Total treatment time is 45 minutes

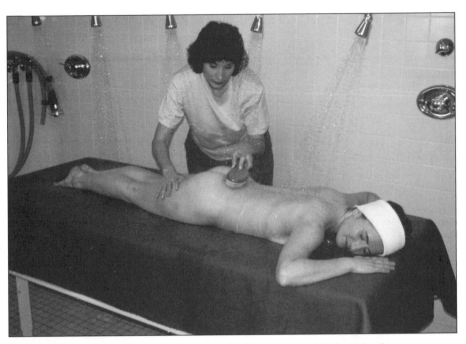

FIGURE 4-4 *Annette Hanson demonstrates a salt glow treatment with the Vichy shower.*

with 15 minutes for cleanup, changeover, sales. The client doesn't turn over, just side to side (Figure 4-4).

Vichy Shower/Mud or Seaweed

Book 45 minutes to 1 1/4 hours, depending on whether the treatments are for the full body or partial body. The wrap time for most muds and seaweeds is 30 minutes. The Vichy shower time will be 10 minutes. The application and completion time will vary according to the area being worked on. Final lotion application may take only a few moments in a spot treatment or about 5–10 minutes for a full body.

Vichy Shower/Salt Glow/Mud or Seaweed

Book 90 minutes. Allow 35 minutes for the salt exfoliation and 20 minutes for the Vichy shower and lotion application. The wrap time is normally 30 minutes but may vary according to the manufacturer. Cleanup, changeover, and sales time is usually the same.

NOTE: *There are other treatment variations available, but these are the most typical. Application time, wrap time, and removal time may vary according to the products. Consult the manufacturer for specifics. Combinations can be fatiguing to the client. Again refer to manufacturer and experience when combining more than two treatments.*

PRICE
Vichy showers range from $2,000 to $5,000.

The Steam Shower

Even though the reference here will be a steam shower, this means also steam cabinets, steam rooms, and steam capability in the actual shower itself—in other words, any environment of moist heat/steam capability. The purpose of steam, as is well known throughout history, is to utilize the heat and moist air to cause the body to perspire, thus facilitating the elimination of toxins, stimulating circulation, and increasing respiration. Some people can't take much steam so steam treatment must be closely watched. The opposite of moist heat, the sauna, will be discussed in chapter 12.

Although the sauna is almost a requirement of the destination spa and health club, it is not often a requirement of the day spa. Most modalities for day spa treatment are more hydrotherapy based. Combining these modalities with the sauna can often be too much for the average client. From a treatment standpoint, it is also more effective to use showers and steam in conjunction with products than with the dry heat of the sauna, which can potentially cause product irritation on the skin.

The steam room, shower, or cabinet is a very popular treatment, from a relaxation standpoint as well as to clear sinuses and respiratory congestion. Warm, moist heat for short periods of time is also great for the skin. However, prolonged time in steam will cause the heat to overpower the moisture and the skin may become dehydrated. When the steam shower, cabinet, or room are used in conjunction with the various showers, it's important to apply hydrating products to the skin during and after treatment. Steam showers, cabinets, or rooms are great to use prior to the body treatment or as a treatment by itself. If the client comes only for the steam then it might be a good idea to be sure that at least a lotion is applied after the steaming to rehydrate the skin and tie product sales to the treatment.

From a cost standpoint, it is more cost effective to have a steam shower than a steam room and it also prevents the client from beginning to equate your day spa with a health club. Your main goal is treatment, not self-relaxation after rigorous exercise. A good modality to follow steam is a cool shower or other showers with cold capabilities unless product application follows. If product application follows, the cool to cold treatment is not recommended at this point unless the client is overheated.

RULES OF THE STEAM SHOWER

- Client should not use immediately after eating.

- The steam shower must be cleaned regularly and no mold can be allowed to grow anywhere.

- If using essential oil infusions in conjunction with the steam, be cautious and keep the amount of infusion quite mild. Steam accelerates the effect on the body. A little goes a long way. Eucalyptus and camphor are commonly used, but be cautious and don't mix with each other or with other essences.

- The time in the steam shower should be kept about the same as the Swiss shower, depending on the treatment following. If the treatment is only the steam, maximum time at about 105 degrees should be 10–15 minutes. Inexperienced and elderly clients should stay in the steam no more than 5–10 minutes.

SAMPLE TREATMENT

1. Client enters spa, undresses, and enters steam shower. If using steam cabinet or room, the client should take a regular cleansing shower first.

2. If the client is getting only the steam shower, it's wise to alternate hot and cold therapy—a few minutes in warm steam, a minute in cool shower—back and forth 2–3 times. Eliminate cool step if the steam shower is a prelude to other treatments.

3. Upon completion of the steam shower, the client either proceeds to the treatment or should be rubbed down with lotion and then counselled on what to do at home.

PRICE

Varies greatly depending on how made, but normally from $1,200 to 2,000.

. . . .

SPA POINT

Do not consider the steam shower as one does in a health club. The steam shower should, in reality, be used in conjunction with another treatment to heighten the effects and to keep it up to the par of a day spa concept.

. . . .

Scotch Hose

Some people refer to the Scotch hose also as a Scots shower, or by some as a Galien jet. They are the same. A Scotch hose is an exciting modality and rather different. The concept behind treatment with a Scotch hose is to target a strong stream of water at specific areas of the body to dramatically increase circulation and elimination and break up fat deposits. The client normally stands next to a wall holding onto handles attached to the wall while the technician shoots water from a device similar to a fire hose from a distance of 8–10 feet away. Some manufacturers have various nozzles and versions that require longer and shorter distances for spraying purposes. Due to the strength of the water pressure and normal distances for treatment, the Scotch hose requires more lengthwise space in a room. It works well in destination spa environments where space is not quite as critical as in a day spa where space may be severely limited. Therefore, in smaller day spas, a Scotch hose may not be practical.

Another way to offer the Scotch hose treatment is to have a large wet room with both the hydrotherapy tub and Scotch hose in the same room. Obviously two different people shouldn't be treated simultaneously, but if the room is free either treatment could be done or a combined treatment could be offered to a single client. This will make the most of the cost of a wet room and the space needed anyway for a hydrotherapy tub. The Scotch hose must be done in a wet room.

RULES OF THE SCOTCH HOSE

- Be sure the water pressure and temperature are not too strong for the client.

- Explain the procedure to the client in advance of treatment so that the client knows you will be in the treatment room while he/she is naked. (If desired, a bathing suit may be worn.)

- Do not be too overaggressive in cellulite treatment. Slight numbness is common for some people after a few minutes. Discontinue treatment at this point or after about 5–10 minutes.

- Do not do a very long treatment on someone who finds standing difficult or weakens easily under water treatment. A person who is not very healthy should be slowly integrated into this treatment beginning with very short periods of time, 5 minutes at the most, gradually increasing as the constitution strengthens.

- If doing in conjunction with a tub treatment, you may want to do a quick Scotch hose before and after the tub. If ending with the Scotch hose, a cool final splash is ideal.

SAMPLE TREATMENT

1. Client removes clothes and enters room. Technician should explain details of the treatment.

2. The technician may choose to shoot water only at the back side or both front and back sides. Client must stand with legs apart for steadiness. Choice of starting on the front side or back side is optional. Sometimes it is preferred to do the front so that the client can relax more when the back side is done. On the other hand, if the client is nervous or hesitant, it's better to do the back side first to relieve the insecurities at the outset and then the client will feel more comfortable about the front side.

3. The client is sprayed overall to relax and warm the entire body. Then with a stronger intensity, warm water should be sprayed at the specific areas of slower metabolism, cellulite, or where you want the water stimulation to take place. The breasts and face should be avoided. The spray may also be guided along with a proper lymph drainage movement, thighs to groin, etc. The length of spray in each area should be no more than 2–3 minutes at most.

4. The hose should be moved from one area to the next and back again so as not to concentrate too long in just one area. The entire duration of the treatment should be about 10–15 minutes at the most.

5. For the experienced or very healthy individual, the treatment may be performed with alternating warm and cool water. Very hot and very cold water should be avoided due to the potential shock to the system. The client should be comfortable at all times.

6. Spraying should take place in a smooth movement from top of the head to the feet if aiming at the back side. If doing the front side, begin with the feet and move up to the shoulders avoiding the breasts and face. If

specifically targeting the stomach and abdominal area, the direction of movement must be in conjunction with the movement of the colon, that is, clockwise. After the overall smooth opening movements, the spray can then be targeted to the areas of concentration. After a few minutes on the concentrated areas, the treatment should end again with a smooth overall spray.

7. Some people also enjoy alternating hot and cold in this treatment as well. If doing both, end the treatment with a quick cold spray to finish on an invigorating note.

8. Be sure the client is steady and feels fine at the end of the treatment before proceeding to the tub or whatever treatment is scheduled next.

PRICES

Scotch hoses may vary from $2,000 to $4,000 depending on the number of hoses and attachments. One hose alone may be sufficient for some needs depending on other modalities available.

BLENDING HYDROTHERAPY MODALITIES

Each device that we've discussed has tremendous assets in the day spa. At least one must be involved to truly call yourself a day spa with hydrotherapy treatments. Water and a sponge in a bowl doesn't really qualify a salon to be a day spa. It doesn't mean that the salon can't start offering body treatments, but the difference in treatment capability is too great to equate the two. Now, the difficulty is choosing which of these devices to put in your day spa. This issue will be dealt with in Day Spa Operations and is a very important one. From a treatment standpoint, you will never use every single device on the same day with any given client any more than does an esthetician use every piece of facial equipment in a facial treatment. The choice depends on the treatment, the client's skin, the time frame, and other variables.

The variables for choosing the equipment are great. Space in an existing salon versus building a brand new day spa is a major consideration. The very least you must have is a plain shower, the very ultimate is the hydrotherapy tub and the rest lie somewhere in between. Please refer to Day Spa Operations and receive guidance from experts in the field on your particular needs.

And finally, the critical issue to your success with hydrotherapy and wet rooms is the sanitary procedures you employ. You absolutely must be immaculate, clean, sanitary. This means someone has to clean and sanitize the room and equipment between every client. You must either hire an assistant for this or be sure your staff understands that this is part of the job. Many technicians want to do treatments but refuse to clean up, or if it's required they get lazy and do a bad job. This can kill your business. Do not forget to deal with this at the hiring of an employee.

. . . .

SPA POINT

There are many exciting devices to choose from, to combine to offer the best in hydrotherapy and real day spa treatment. The choice and development of treatments is based upon budget and many other factors. The most important factor, however, is the cleanliness and sanitary practices of the spa. An unclean wet room will kill the business without you even realizing it.

. . . .

Synopsis

As has been demonstrated, water therapy is the crux of the day spa along with body treatments. From the basic shower to the most sophisticated Vichy shower, the opportunity and convenience of having these tools serve to enhance the effectiveness of every treatment offered in the spa. They further serve to save time, energy, and effort on the part of the technician when it comes to efficacy of treatment and cleaning. With most product lines, you can wash the product off with a sponge and bowl of water; it's just not terribly efficient and takes a great deal more time. The time conservation alone in a short time will more than pay the cost of the installation of the equipment. It is also the opinion of this author that you must be a professional in whatever you do. The showers at least keep you on the cutting edge of professionalism. And finally, not to beat it to death, but the cleaning and sanitation of the showers is tantamount to your success. If there is ever even a hint of a question in a client's mind about whether they might pick up a virus or disease you're on your way out of business. You can't let the thought even arise and to avoid the problem, extreme sanitation is preferable.

Review

1. Why is a shower important in a day spa?
2. What is the difference between a regular shower and a Swiss shower?
3. Can a Vichy shower treatment be done by itself? Is it a good idea? Why?
4. What is the benefit of a steam shower/cabinet/room?
5. What types of treatments work well with a Vichy shower?
6. What is a Scotch hose? For what is it used?
7. Why is good sanitation so important with hydrotherapy?

CHAPTER 5
Touch and Massage _____

OVERVIEW

In order to do body treatments, the ideal situation is to be fully trained in the art of body massage. Depending on the state, a massage therapist license may also be necessary to do any type of body treatments. It is the responsibility of the technician to find out and obey all applicable laws.

For the sake of this book, a short introduction to massage concepts is important for the person intending to do day spa body treatments and to gain the trust and confidence of the client. It's obviously necessary also for the effective application of body products in treatments.

As has already been discussed in great detail, the novice client to body treatment needs as much reassurance as possible in order to get beyond the shyness of body care. A good sense of touch properly placed at the outset of treatment will go a long way in relaxing and reassuring the client. Let's look at how this mechanism of touch can help.

MECHANISM OF TOUCH

It's interesting to just consider how we use the word *touch* in our normal everyday vocabulary. "Isn't that touching?" "I'm touched by what you said." "What a soft touch." "The flowers made a perfect added touch to the look." "She seems so untouchable." Sometimes we don't realize how much the word alone impacts our lives.

When it comes to the subject of touch in general, we so often overlook the profound impact it has on us all. In the next few paragraphs, I will be excerpting information from a book called *The Gift of the Blessing*, by Gary Smalley and John Trent, Ph.D., published by Thomas Nelson Publishers.

"A little four-year-old girl became frightened late one night during a thunderstorm. After one particularly loud clap of thunder, she jumped from her bed, ran down the hall, and burst into her parents' room. Jumping right into the middle of the bed, she sought out her parents' arms for comfort and assurance. 'Don't worry, Honey,' her father said, trying to calm her fears. 'The Lord will protect you.' The little girl snuggled closer to her father and said, 'I know that, Daddy, but right now I need someone with skin on.'"

From the physiological standpoint, tremendous research has been done in recent years on the effect of touch or massage on the human body and mind. According to authors Smalley and Trent, a Dr. Dolores Kreiger, professor of nursing at New York University, did a number of studies on the effects of touch and revealed that the hemoglobin levels of both the patient and person touching go up during touch. As the hemoglobin levels go up, the body tissues receive more oxygen and the person is energized. Almost everyone is now aware that residents of nursing homes who have pets to touch and hold have been shown to live longer and have better attitudes than those without, clearly demonstrating another positive effect of touch.

Another interesting example cited in Smalley and Trent's book is of interest. "A doctor we know, a noted neurosurgeon, did his own study on the effects of brief times of touch. With half his patients in the hospital, he would sit on their bed and touch them on the arm or leg when he came in to see how they were doing. With his remaining patients, he would simply stand near the bed to conduct his interview of how they were feeling. Before the patients went home from the hospital, the nurses gave each patient a short questionnaire evaluating the treatment they received. They were especially asked to comment on the amount of time they felt the doctor had spent with them. While in actuality he had spent the same amount of time in each patient's room, those people he had sat down near and touched felt he had been in their room nearly twice as long as those he had not touched."

· ·

SPA POINT

We don't consider how influential the entire subject of touch is in our lives today. The emotional and physical impact on each of us is tremendous. The properly placed touch can work wonders in relaxing a client, relieving stress, and creating a sense of well-being. Touch is the foundation of a successful day spa.

· ·

HISTORY

Now, let's take a brief look at history. Hippocrates, the Father of Medicine, used massage extensively in healing, and touch, as in the "laying on of hands" and "anointing" the body with potions and creams, has existed for nearly five thousand years. Touch is discussed numerous times in the Bible and is still an important part of many religious practices today. The people of ancient civilizations of Egypt, Rome, Greece, China, and Japan have all used some form of massage and touch to apply oils, creams, unguents, and perfumes not only to beautify the body but also to embalm the dead. Ancient Romans had slaves carry oils in glass containers slung over their arms to massage their masters on call.

During the course of history massage also had its times of popularity and times when it fell almost into oblivion. With time and progress also came confusion about massage and the methodology. Peter Henry Ling of Sweden (1776–1839) probably made the greatest modern impact on massage development the world had seen up to that time. He is credited with developing a systematic approach to massage that ultimately became the internationally known Swedish System of Massage that we practice to this very day. His system of massage introduced terms such as effleurage, petrissage, friction, vibration, as well as rolling, pinching, and several other descriptions. But it still wasn't until the end of the nineteenth century that massage began to really be favored and accepted worldwide. Dr. Mezger of

Holland (1839–1901) helped achieve reputable recognition for massage in England and parts of America. By 1900 in England, massage was finally licensed by the Board of Trade, and organizations regulating it were formed.

In America, however, the relevance of massage has been hard in coming. Over the last two hundred years, massage was predominantly practiced by women of ill repute and opportunists. On the respectable side, it seemed to stay under the purview of the physiotherapist in a clinical setting. Fortunately, over the last couple of decades massage has finally begun to gain recognition as a viable relaxation and well-being therapy for all Americans. Massage therapy organizations and licensure has finally begun to take place in most states, and the public no longer scoffs at the idea of getting a massage. There are currently a number of research projects being sponsored by the National Institutes of Health to further ascertain the benefits of massage. By looking back on history, we can see how long this practice has been a viable part of our society. The trick now is to bring it to common usage in beauty and health maintenance for all people everywhere.

Touch and the Skin

To better understand the mechanism of the skin and touch sensation, the following is excerpted from my book published by Milady Publishing Company, *Shiatsu Massage*.

Without making this a text on the anatomy and physiology of the skin, it's useful to consider the skin and its relationship to massage, not only from the client's standpoint but from the technician's as well. Amma massage in Japan was originally based upon the idea that a blind person was best suited to massage because of the superior refinement of the sense of touch. Touch is integral to the success of Shiatsu for both giver and receiver.

Consider for a moment how complex the largest organ of the body, the skin, is:

According to *Milady's Standard Textbook for Professional Estheticians*, one square inch of skin contains:

- 65 hairs
- 95–100 sebaceous glands
- 78 yards of nerves
- 19 yards of blood vessels
- 650 sweat glands
- 9,500,000 cells
- 1,300 nerve endings to record pain
- 19,500 sensory cells at the ends of nerve fibers
- 78 sensory apparatuses for heat
- 13 sensory apparatuses for cold

• 160–165 pressure apparatuses for perception of tactile stimuli

There are sensory nerve fibers in the skin that react to four basic sensations: pressure, touch, temperature (heat and cold), and pain. The sensory aspect of the skin is what we deal with most in understanding how and where the technician is to use pressure to perform the treatment and also to understand the comfort and response levels of the client.

Within the skin are different sensory receptors that record the different sensations, many of them named after the scientists who found them. There are:

1. Free nerve endings—pain receptors from the many branches of nerves.

2. Ruffini endings—notably heat receptors.

3. Pacinian corpuscle—encapsulated endings normally located between the dermis and subcutaneous layers that are receptors for deeper pressure.

4. Meissner's corpuscles—common receptors for light touch that are located in the dermis.

5. Krause's corpuscles—heat receptors located in the upper area of the dermis.

The previous relates to these receptors at skin level. In the deeper parts of the body, such as the muscles and joints, the roles may be different or overlap to a degree, and the additional Golgi tendon organ in muscle tendons responds to provide information on contraction, muscle stretch, and passive and active tension of the muscle.

· ·

SPA POINT

With so many receptors in and on our skin, the importance of massage and touch cannot be overemphasized. The client and technician as well will physically benefit from massage.

· ·

EFFECTS OF MASSAGE

From a purely practical standpoint and from a marketing standpoint, what will massage do for the client? What are the benefits of massage that will further facilitate the effects of body treatments with products? Massage…

… causes an increase in the blood circulation and helps to improve overall nutritional exchanges in the body.

… improves the body's own metabolism to facilitate absorption of nutrition and elimination of wastes and toxins.

… can help relieve soreness and discomfort in muscles.

… can help relieve mental and physical fatigue.

… has a sedative effect on the nervous system and relaxes, thus reducing stress.

… feels good and gives the client a sense of well-being.

… improves skin texture and softness.

Client Consultation Prior to Treatment

Now, before beginning any treatment, it's important to talk with the client. You must know if the client is having a treatment for the first time or is experienced. This will be a critical factor in the client's comfort level. If it's the first time, you must discuss the fact that the client will be completely covered and only the part of the body actually being worked on will be exposed. Whether it be a massage or a body treatment, it's important to keep a few things in mind.

- The client must be instructed on how to undress, what robe to put on, how to lie on the table (face up or down and at which end of the bed).

- Contraindications of treatment must be determined before the treatment begins.

- Client comfort and warmth is critical. Be sure to ask.

- Comfortable touch and pressure should be determined several times near the beginning of the treatment.

- If possible and equipment is available, have the client shower before the treatment begins. This will not only ensure cleanliness but also warm and begin to relax the muscles.

. . . .

SPA POINT

Massage is an overall wellness and feel-better concept because the massage itself can stimulate metabolism and blood circulation to increase nutrition and release toxins and wastes from the body more efficiently.

. . . .

Contraindications to Massage

Keep in mind that there may be a large difference in the contraindications when doing a full massage versus using some effleurage (gentle stroking) to begin the application of products for a body treatment. Contraindications for body treatment in general and for specific treatments will be more fully discussed in another chapter. There are some contraindications that should be mentioned for simple massage as well.

- Do not apply pressure to any vascularized areas such as distended capillaries in the face or varicose veins on the legs or other parts of the body.

- Do not do massage when the health of the client is in question, particularly in cases of cancer, HIV active status, or any other chronic systemic disease. Be sure to obtain a physician's written release to perform treatment.

- Do not massage areas of open wounds, infection, inflammation, lumps or bumps, or swelling.

- Do not massage a client who is pregnant, particularly the abdomen, without specific training in dealing with pregnancy.

- Do not massage in any situation when in doubt.

NOTE: *Doing massage on the opposite sex may be determined by state or local statute. If it is not, use cautious judgment when performing massage on a stranger in an environment where you might be alone. In many cases it is better not to do a massage on a stranger. Or, you may choose to have someone with you on premises during that time.*

· ·

SPA POINT

Massage should never be done on anyone but a normally healthy person. Chronic disease, inflammation, swelling, systemic disease, vascular issues, and anything questionable are always contraindicated for massage.

· ·

THE CLASSICAL EFFLEURAGE MASSAGE

As you will learn in a full course on massage, traditional Swedish massage will include a number of movements. For this book, however, we will concentrate on effleurage as it's the movement of choice in opening a body treatment and for product application.

The purpose of effleurage is to open the treatment with a gentle touch in a soft stroking movement. Strong pressure is not desired in the opening of a treatment. For simplicity of understanding, Swedish effleurage massage is generally performed toward the heart. That is to say, for example, when doing the legs, the stroking will take place from the foot upward toward the groin. Massage for the arms will likewise be from the hand to the axilla (armpit).

Assuming for a moment that you will be doing a full-body massage, there are several schools of thought on where to begin and end the massage. There are no hard and fast rules and often it is merely a matter of choice. Some technicians like to massage the front of the body first to gain the client's trust and begin the relaxation process so that by the time the back is done, the client will be completely relaxed. Others believe that it's better to do the back first to more quickly gain client confidence and relaxation. Either is fine, but for this book, the front of the body will be done first. It is also important to know that depending on the body treatment being performed, the order and approach may be quite different. For example, in a full-body massage, once the front side is done, the client is asked to roll over onto the stomach. When doing a slippery mud or seaweed treatment, however, the client is not asked to completely roll over due to potential for the client to slip off the bed. So the order of movement from one part to the next will vary as will be shown later. But for now, considering massage only, the following gives a good general flow of one part to the other.

Order of Massage

Client is lying on back with head at the front of the bed or table.

1. Foot of one leg.
2. Move from foot to calf, knee, thigh.
3. Move to other leg, do foot, calf, knee, thigh.
4. Move to hand on same side of body.
5. Move from hand to lower arm, elbow, upper arm.
6. Move to other hand and do hand, lower arm, elbow, upper arm.
7. Move to top of head if doing head. If doing head, do massage on scalp then face. Then move to chest.
8. If not doing head, move from arm to chest. Massage chest.
9. Massage back of neck.
10. If desired and preferred by client, perform gentle massage on stomach in clockwise direction only and upward from lower abdomen to just below rib cage.

Client now rolls over onto stomach.

1. Again repeat back of one leg from foot to buttocks.
2. Do other leg.
3. Normally arms are not done again, but do back of arms if desired.
4. Move to top of head and perform massage on scalp if applicable.
5. Massage back of neck again.
6. Massage back.
7. Massage upper buttocks if applicable.

Performance of Massage in Relation to Body Treatments

Since this is not a book on massage, we will not go into muscles, origin and insertion of muscles, or the skeletal structure. As stated at the beginning, all body treatments will be better with more knowledge. Taking a course in body massage is very important, whether it's a short crash course or a full licensing course. If you're an esthetician and have been trained in facial massage, the premise is the same. Open with effleurage and then proceed to the next step. However, there are some large differences between facial and body treatment.

- Pressure to the area being massaged should come from the shoulders and body of the technician.

- Use full hands and mold hands to the part of the body being massaged. Do not employ just the fingertips as you would in some facial massage.

- Use long full-flowing movements on any area being worked on. Larger movements are preferable on the body.

- On large areas such as the back, the technician should rock his or her own body into the rhythm of the movement.

- You must use more pressure in effleurage on the body than in for the face, but not so heavy as to feel uncomfortable for the client.

· ·

SPA POINT

Effleurage is a gentle stroking manipulation that will be used in all body treatments for exfoliation and application of products. Students should master the effleurage technique before complicating treatment with products and hydrotherapy. This is the aspect of any treatment that wins and holds the client.

· ·

General Effleurage for the Body

PROCEDURE

1. Beginning with one foot, alternate strokes up, over, and around the foot (Figure 5-1).

2. Effleurage up and down sole of foot and then up and down Achilles tendon (behind ankle) (Figure 5-2).

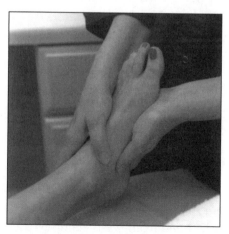 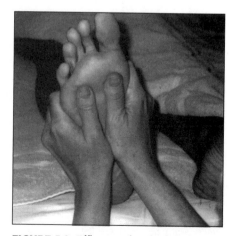

FIGURE 5-1 *Alternate strokes around the foot.*   FIGURE 5-2 *Effleurage the sole of the foot.*

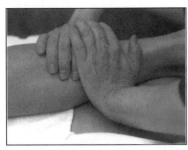

FIGURE 5-3 *With hands overlapped, stroke up the front of the calf.*

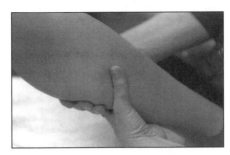

FIGURE 5-4 *Stroke the back of the calf.*

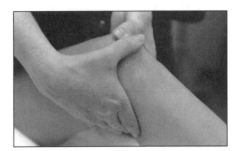

FIGURE 5-5 *Using thumbs, circle the knee.*

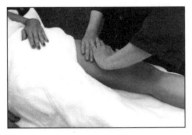

FIGURE 5-6 *Overlap hands and stoke up the leg, from the knee to the thigh.*

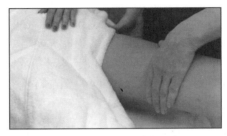

FIGURE 5-7 *Stroke the inside of the thigh.*

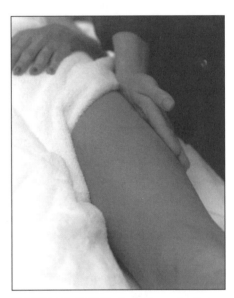

FIGURE 5-8 *With the back of your hand, stroke the outside of the thigh.*

3. Overlap hands and stroke up the front of the calf (Figure 5-3). Then alternate hands and lift leg to stroke up the back of the calf (Figure 5-4).

4. Use thumbs to circle the knee about three times (Figure 5-5).

5. Overlap hands and stroke from knee to top of thigh on the top (Figure 5-6), then use one hand for support while other hand strokes the inside thigh (Figure 5-7) and outside thigh (Figure 5-8).

6. Move to other leg and repeat steps 1–5.

7. Move to arm on same side as leg just massaged. Stroke outside and inside of hands (Figure 5-9).

8. Support arm and let other hand stroke from wrist to top of arm (Figure 5-10), circling the elbow. While one hand supports, the other hand alternates effleurage on the inside and outside of the upper arm (Figure 5-11).

9. Move to other arm and repeat steps 7–8.

10. If doing head, use the fingers of both hands to gently stroke the scalp from the forehead to the crown (Figure 5-12). Lift head slightly to then stroke head from the base up to the crown. Do several rows as necessary to complete head.

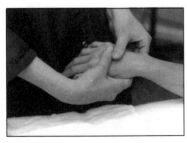

FIGURE 5-9 *Using thumbs and fingers, stroke the inside and the outside of the hands.*

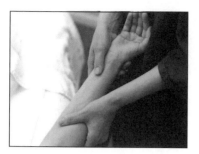

FIGURE 5-10 *Stroke from the wrist to the top of the arm.*

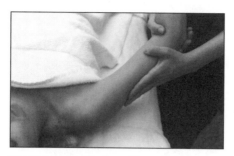

FIGURE 5-11 *Alternate effleurage on the inside and outside of the upper arm.*

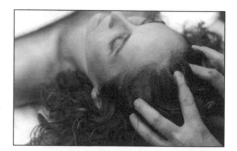

FIGURE 5-12 *Gently stroke the head, from the forehead to the crown.*

11. If doing face, do effleurage as always done in facial massage.

12. If not doing head or face, delete steps 10–11. Move from arm to chest.

13. At the center of the chest just below the clavicle (collarbone), gently make circular motions with both hands from the sternum (center) out to the axilla (armpit). This should be repeated in rows from the clavicle down to just above the nipple area (Figure 5-13).

14. Slide around shoulders and glide up and down back of neck and upper shoulders several times. The massage at this point may end off the shoulders or earlobes.

15. Massage of the stomach/abdomen is optional. If doing stomach, be sure strokes go from the lower abdomen upward and outward (Figure 5-14). No movement should go counterclockwise in order to maintain proper directional flow to colon.

Client turns over onto stomach and the back side begins.

1. Beginning with same leg as previously, this time overlap hands and glide from the ankle straight up the leg to the top of the leg just below the buttocks. Reduce pressure at the point of the back of the knee as this area is very delicate. The thigh will be done as on the front. After the center row, one hand will support and one hand will glide up the inside and outside of the thigh (Figure 5-15).

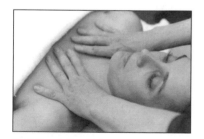

FIGURE 5-13 *With circular motions, massage the chest; avoid the nipple area.*

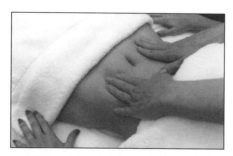

FIGURE 5-14 *Stroke the stomach from the lower abdomen upward and outward.*

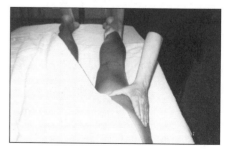

FIGURE 5-15 *Using one hand, glide up the inside and outside of the thigh.*

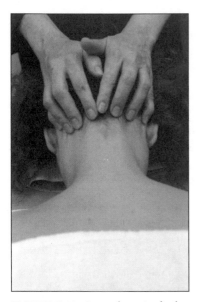

FIGURE 5-16 *Cover the entire back of the head with massage. Fingers should glide from base of the head to top of the head.*

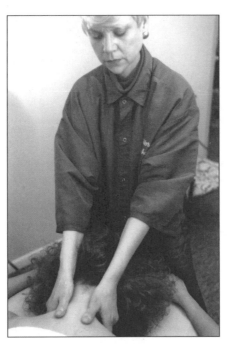

FIGURE 5-17 *Massage the back of the neck.*

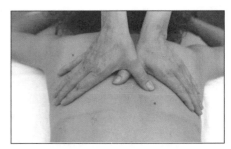

FIGURE 5-18 *With full hands, glide down the center of the back with thumbs on opposite sides of the spine.*

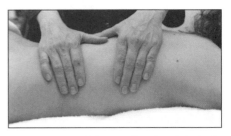

FIGURE 5-19 *Glide over the sides of the back.*

2. Repeat other leg.

3. Normally arms are not done again, but if desired do stroking movement in similar manner as on the back of the legs. Do not lift arms off table.

4. If doing head again, allow fingers to glide from base of head to top of head in several rows to cover entire back of head (Figure 5-16).

5. Slide up back of neck several times (Figure 5-17).

6. The back has several movements. Begin with full hands gliding down the center of back with thumbs on opposite sides of spine (Figure 5-18). Glide to base of back and slide out to the sides and back up to top of shoulders, out over the tops of the arms and back to the center of the trapezius (muscle at top of back in center) at the base of the neck. Then alternating hands, glide over the entire sides of the back (Figure 5-19). This can be done from a position at the head or by going to the side of the bed. Then for the other side of the back, move to the other side of the bed. Then once again slide down the back and up the sides.

7. If desired and appropriate for the client, massage may be performed on the upper buttocks. Firm pressure should be applied as hands glide across the upper buttocks in a circular motion (Figure 5-20). Do not allow the areas to flop around. Less movement of the cheeks of the buttocks is most comfortable for the client. Finally slide from the buttocks back up to the top of the back and off the shoulders.

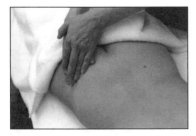

FIGURE 5-20 *With firm pressure, glide hands across the upper buttocks in a circular motion.*

Synopsis

Unless you're a massage therapist, you won't be performing a massage that flows from one movement to the next as described, but the actual movements on each body part are quite applicable to any body treatment, including exfoliating procedures. A big difference in a body treatment where a wrap is used will be wrapping two legs together first and then moving up the body. This will be somewhat different as you will see later. Practicing smooth movements and transitions from one place to another will definitely help you develop a good sense of touch and proficiency when it comes to adding treatments and hydrotherapy. The ability to perform all body treatments will be contingent upon smooth handling of the body as in the massage discussed previously. Also, there is deliberately no mention of other massage movements such as vibration or kneading, as these movements are not normally related to a body treatment.

Review

1. What is so important about touch?
2. What has research shown massage to do for both the technician and receiver?
3. Who is considered to be the Father of Modern Massage?
4. Why has respectability for massage been hard in coming in America?
5. What are two effects of massage?
6. Why is client consultation important before a treatment?
7. What is a common contraindication for massage?
8. What type of movement will be used for massage as done in conjunction with body treatments?

CHAPTER 6
Introduction to Aromatherapy

DISCLAIMER: PLEASE BE AWARE THAT THIS CHAPTER IS PURELY AN INTRODUCTION TO AROMATHERAPY. THE SCOPE OF TRUE AROMATHERAPY GOES FAR BEYOND THE SIMPLICITY OF THIS CHAPTER, WHICH IS DESIGNED TO OPEN THE STUDENT'S EYES SOME, FACILITATE A PRACTICAL APPLICATION OF CERTAIN OILS, AND STIMULATE FURTHER STUDY. PLEASE REFER TO SALONOVATION'S GUIDE TO AROMATHERAPY, BY SHELLEY HESS, ALONG WITH JOEL GERSON'S STANDARD TEXTBOOK FOR PROFESSIONAL ESTHETICIANS.

OVERVIEW

Aromatherapy, an ancient art and science but still new and exciting today, plays a large role in the beauty industry in general but particularly in day spa treatments. The word *aromatherapy* means the therapeutic use of aromatic essences from plants in treatment for beauty and well-being (Figure 6-1). Even though aromatherapy concepts are new to many, the practice may date as far back as five thousand years.

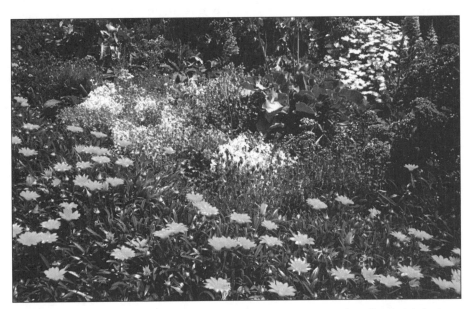

FIGURE 6-1 *The aromatic essences used in aromatherapy treatments are from flower and plant extractions.*

HISTORY

The ancient Egyptians and Romans are renowned for their usage of essential oils in medicine and in the bath. Consider Cleopatra and her baths; Hippocrates, who has been credited with using more than three hundred plants in his cures along with massage; or perhaps the famous story of the

Three Wise Men bringing gifts of gold, frankincense, and myrrh to celebrate the birth of the Messiah, Jesus Christ. Frankincense and myrrh are both highly effective essential oils and were valued in Christ's time with gold or any other precious material. We have many references to the anointing with oils throughout the Bible, such as John 12:3, "Mary, therefore took a pound of very costly perfume of pure nard, and anointed the feet of Jesus, and wiped His feet with her hair; and the house was filled with the fragrance of the perfume."

The ancient civilizations highly valued essential oils (aromatic plants perhaps) and used them for medicinal purposes, for embalming the dead, and for personal grooming. There were still remnants of perfume in containers buried in the famous tomb of King Tut when it was opened in the early 1920s. How could a perfume last three thousand years? Much is still to be learned about the preservation and processing of essential oils from thousands of years ago.

Modern Development

Skipping a couple of thousand years or so, the modern development of aromatherapy is quite interesting. We believe the term *aromatherapy* was coined by the famous French perfumer Maurice Gattefosse, who also wrote a book entitled *Aromathérapie* published in 1928. He appears to be the originator of not only the word but also the practice of aromatherapy. Until the 1960s very little had been written about this subject since the 1930s. Dr. Jean Valnet in his 1964 book, *The Practice of Aromatherapy* (English translation of *aromathérapie*) began to develop the concepts and practices of aromatherapy as we use it today by treating war wounds on soldiers in World War II. Today we must credit a number of pioneers who in recent decades have brought aromatherapy to the great prominence it holds in beauty therapy. Most of our knowledge and expertise has come to us from England by experts such as Robert Tisserand (author of excellent aromatherapy books such as *The Art of Aromatherapy*), Micheline Arcier, Eve Taylor, Elisabeth Jones, and Shirley Price. Today, thanks to these and many other people, aromatherapy is the most popular modality in natural treatment for the face and body. Now, let's consider what it is.

• •

SPA POINT

History shows us the importance of essential oils. If an essence can be used to mummify a person and still have a scent three thousand years later, there must be something important about aromatherapy.

• •

ESSENTIAL OILS

Perhaps the word used for the extracts from plants, essential oil, was chosen because what is used is the very heart and soul of the plant, or because they were considered to be essential to life, the "essence" of the plant. Es-

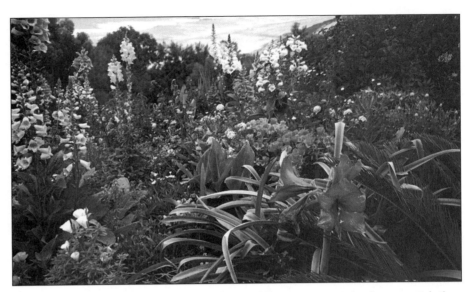

FIGURE 6-2 *The very heart and soul of the plants and flowers are extracted to form essential oils.*

sences may come from the flowers, stems, leaves, root, bark, or even the entire plant (Figure 6-2). These essences are extracted by a variety of techniques that allow the purest, most aromatic essence to be used for perfumes, in aromatherapy, and in herbal medicine.

In many cases we don't really appreciate what it takes to get an essential oil. For example, Bulgarian rose oil is probably the most expensive in the world at more than $1,000 per ounce. It takes thirty roses to make one drop of the oil or sixty thousand petals per ounce. Jasmine, another expensive extract, requires eight million blossoms to get a two-pound yield. When you see highly sophisticated perfumes and wonder why they're so expensive, the answer is predominantly in the raw material cost. A couple of traditional examples are Joy, originally the world's most expensive perfume, which is primarily rose and jasmine. Chanel No. 5 is rose, jasmine, and vanilla. The flowers and plants have to be selected and processed at specific times of the day, month, and year, and the soil, area, country, weather, and climate are all considered. In actuality, the quality variation of essences is really quite similar to that of the myriad of wines. There are hundreds, perhaps as many as 600–800, of essences used today in perfumes, aromatherapy, and medicine.

. . . .

SPA POINT

The "essence" of an essential oil is the life force of that ingredient, the most important part of it (Figure 6-3).

. . . .

Processing Essential Oils

DISTILLATION

Hot steam passes through the plant material causing the essential oil to separate and evaporate along with the water. After the distillant is cooled, the essential oil is usually floating on the surface and can be separated

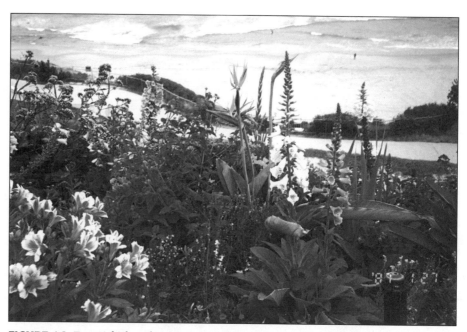

FIGURE 6-3 *Essential oils and water mix well to form a beneficial treatment for your client.*

easily. The remaining distillate water is further saturated with the essential oil to make toilet water. Examples: rose, orange flower.

SOLVENT EXTRACTION
Essences extracted through this process are called *absolutes*. The plants are mixed with a solvent and heated until the essence is dissolved in the solvent. The solution is filtered leaving the essence behind. It is further processed with alcohol to obtain the absolute. Certain flowers and plants are much better processed by this method due to the low heat factor. Example: mimosa, benzoin.

EXPRESSION
This technique cold presses the oils out of a fruit or plant. The essence is collected in a sponge and then squeezed out. Examples: citrus fruits.

ENFLEURAGE
This method is old and only used in very delicate situations. The flower petals are spread across glass plates that have been covered with fat. The plates are stacked and left for 24–48 hours, then replaced with more petals until the fat is saturated. Then an alcohol solvent separates the fat and essence. This process is very slow and can take up to a month or two. Example: tuberose.

MACERATION
This method is similar to enfleurage but the flower petals or other parts of the plant are saturated in hot fat instead of cold fat and then extracted. Examples: various flowers.

How Essential Oils Work

The effect of essential oils on humans is a complicated and not completely understood phenomenon. Yet we know that plant essences can have a powerful, wonderful, and even toxic effect on the body depending on what and how much is used. Essential oils affect the body in two predominant ways, physiologically and psychologically. Physiologically essential oils can affect the person through a number of applications: by ingestion (never recommended in our industry), by infusions (use of a room diffuser), by bathing, with compresses, and through topical massage of the skin. Essential oils are lipophilic (attracted to oil) and have a natural affinity to the skin. They are also normally very small in molecular size and can penetrate the skin easily. For people who tend to disbelieve the theory of results from a topical application, try rubbing garlic oil on a person's feet. Wait half to three-quarters of an hour and you should be able to detect the odor on the breath of that person. It is generally accepted that essential oils are highly penetrative and, as such, have a profound effect on the body. As a result, they are often used as curatives in holistic medicine. Even though the scope of this book is not for medical or curative purposes, it's interesting to note how essential oils can affect the system.

ACTION OF ESSENTIAL OILS

On Skin
They can dissolve dead surface cells, increase cell turnover, stimulate metabolism, improve texture, add softness, give radiance, stimulate and tone.

On Nervous System
They can calm, soothe nerve endings, cause a sense of euphoria, relax.

On Glands
They have a soothing and sedative effect, toning and stimulating; they normalize glandular function.

On Muscles
They can relieve fatigue, reduce soreness and stiffness, improve resistance and elasticity of muscle.

On Blood and Lymph
They can facilitate smooth flow, increase metabolism and elimination of wastes.

In other words, essential oils can, and do, affect the entire body. It's imperative that you understand that they can also be toxic if too much is used or for too long. The psychological effect is also physical to some degree and quite interesting.

. . . .

SPA POINT

We know that essential oils have a powerful effect on the body. Garlic can be rubbed on the feet and then detected in the breath in about 30 minutes.

. . . .

Psychology and the Nose

The sense of smell is controlled by the olfactory system and is perhaps the closest direct link between the brain and the stimulant than the other senses. Olfactory stimulation has the capacity to produce an immediate effect on the nervous system. Any stimulation affects the limbic system, the part of the brain that controls emotions and personality. This also affects the pituitary and other glandular systems. Essences may also play a role in stimulating the production of neurochemicals such as endorphins and enkephalins, the body's own pain killers and relaxants.

It's interesting to note that we have an almost immediate reaction to odors, good and bad. Good odors stay with us throughout our lives. Do you ever remember experiencing a specific fragrance, perhaps your grandmother's perfume, and anytime you smell it, even years later, you instinctively think of your grandmother? Bad odors cause immediate revulsion. Fragrance is such a strong part of our lives, that our moods can be altered with fragrance, some calm us and some excite us. Some fragrances are sensual, and some give us a feeling of relaxation. There are manufacturers of unusual items, such as scented stockings for women (Kanebo Cosmetics, Tokyo), aroma discs, air fresheners, auto fresheners, and others.

Although we don't entirely understand how this all works on us, the fact remains that it does. Essential oils can and do have a profound effect on our personalities. Research continues to be done throughout the world to investigate the power of odor on our psyche right alongside research into the physiological effects of aromatherapy. From a practical standpoint, there will be some confusion to the novice on what oils to combine for what effects and understanding the blends comes only with time and experience. Keep in mind that you're dealing with hundreds of oils and, hence, endless combinations of them. In the next section, we'll discuss some of the more common essences and their uses.

· ·

SPA POINT

Tremendous research is being conducted on the psychological effects fragrances have on us. We know a great perfume on the opposite sex entices us; we use air fresheners to refresh the room; and scents can remind us of friends, events of the past. They have the ability to penetrate our memory and evoke feelings.

· ·

SPA POINT

As is obvious by looking at the history and properties of essential oils, they have survived the test of time, thus having a viable place in the repertoire of the professional. A lifetime of study can be given to this field alone. The main value of incorporating aromatherapy into day spa treatments is to tap into the many and varied effects aromatherapy has on the body, not just from a skin standpoint but also from an overall wellness standpoint, both physically and emotionally. The ambiance that can be created by diffusing the right oils into the air of the treatment room can go far in relaxing and restoring the client, long before the treatment even begins. As such, aromatherapy is a valuable asset in the spa concept.

With research progressing as it is, in the future we may see perfumes that ease stress, strawberry essences in hospital corridors, movies with appropriate fragrances. From a purely treatment standpoint, there's no question that different essences can have direct impact on the body, from chamomile for soothing skin to rosemary as a stimulant. As with all subjects, and perhaps more so with aromatherapy, do not attempt to play doctor and cure people of ailments. This is not under the purview of our licensure and could serve to injure the entire industry in the future.

. . . .

Some Common Essential Oils and Their Purposes

The variety and mix of essential oils is probably the most intimidating aspect of aromatherapy. There are oils with top notes, midnotes, base notes. There are oils of yin and yang quality. There are oils that are considered to be stimulating or sedative or sometimes both. What oils do is rather subjective and depends to a great extent on the expertise of the practitioner. As frustrating as this may be to the beginner, it's also exciting to know that in this subject alone you can continue to experiment and grow for many years to come. Just as no two hairdressers cut the same head of hair the same way, no two aromatherapy experts will necessarily agree on combinations.

The following oils were chosen for general use purposes and are in no way the only oils out there for you to use. Next to the name of the oil you will see any number of purposes listed. Some include medical reference points, not for you to practice medicine but purely from an informational point of view.

Basil (herb):	Antistress, antiseptic, toning.
Benzoin (gum):	Antiseptic, sedative, euphoric.
Bergamot (fruit):	Antiacne, good for psoriasis and excema, antiseptic, healing, deodorizing, helps fight infection, uplifting. (Caution: use 1 percent or less due to photosensitivity; do not expose to sun.)
Birch (bark):	Astringent, similar to wintergreen, reduces soreness and stiffness of muscles and joints.
Camphor (wood):	Stimulates and soothes, cools then heats, stimulates heart, analgesic, antiseptic, rubefacient, stimulates circulation, can be vasoconstrictor. (Caution: overuse can be toxic.)
Cedarwood (wood):	Antiseptic, astringent, sedative, good for skin eruptions/psoriasis/excema/seborrhea.
Chamomile (flower):	Calms nerves, sedative, soothes inflammations, reduces stress, antidepressant, good for burns, antiseptic, analgesic, derivative azulene (colorant and soothing agent), antiallergenic, may reduce

body temperature. Known also as the "plant's physician" because it keeps other plants healthy.

Cinnamon (herb): Antiseptic, stimulant, warming. (Caution: must dilute.)

Clary sage (herb): Antidepressant, relaxant, antiseptic, calms, euphoric, warms, sedative. (Caution: can intoxicate.)

Clove (flower bud): Analgesic, antiseptic, stimulant, strengthens memory, soothes muscles. (Caution: must dilute.)

Cypress (fruit): Vasoconstrictor, antiseptic, astringent, sedative, good for varicose veins, similar effect as juniper and pine.

Eucalyptus (leaves): One of the best antiseptics, disinfectant, analgesic, astringent, rubefacient, good for muscle soreness, pronounced cooling effect on body, excellent on fever, decongestant.

Fennel (seeds): Antiseptic, toning, diuretic.

Frankincense (gum): Antiseptic, calming, astringent, sedative, warming, toning, slightly anti-inflammatory, rejuvenating.

Geranium (herb): Anti-inflammatory, enhances relaxation, analgesic, antiseptic, sedative, blends well with other oils, reduces anxiety, uplifting.

Grapefruit (fruit): Astringent, cleansing, stimulant, toning, anticellulite/water retention.

Jasmine (flower): Soothing, relaxing, antiseptic, antidepressant, slightly anti-inflammatory, considered "king" of flowers, very expensive.

Juniper (fruit): Astringent, antiseptic, invigorating, toning, antitoxic, rubefacient, both stimulating and relaxing, stimulates circulation, diuretic.

Lavender (flower): Antiseptic, relaxant, analgesic, antitoxic, diuretic, sudorific, reduces inflammation, very cleansing/purifying/calming, antistress, soothes burns, antiacne. Considered the most useful and versatile.

Lemon (fruit): Antiseptic, bactericidal, detoxifies, purifies.

Lemongrass (herb): Antiseptic, purifying, great for oily hair and skin, sedative, stimulating. (Caution: quite strong, use diluted.)

Melissa (herb):	Antiseptic, antidepressant, relaxes, reduces stress, sedative, antiallergenic.
Myrrh (gum):	Antiseptic, astringent, sedative, toning, purifies, reduces inflammation, cools skin, antiaging.
Neroli (flower):	Antidepressant, calming, facial softener, sedative, nonirritating, great for redness and inflammation, induces calm. (From bitter orange, *Citrus vulgaris*, not to be confused with sweet orange oil.)
Sweet orange (flower):	Calming, soothing, reduces nervousness, revives complexion.
Oregano (herb):	Antiseptic, analgesic, muscle relaxant, stimulant, energizes.
Patchouli (herb):	Antiseptic, antidepressant, sedative, nerve stimulant, rejuvenating, similar to myrrh, good for dry skin.
Peppermint (herb):	Antiseptic, analgesic, cooling, sedative, antibacterial, vasoconstrictor, main constituent is menthol.
Pine (wood):	Antiseptic, reduces fatigue, reduces muscle stiffness, great for bath.
Rose (flower):	Antiseptic, astringent, sedative, relieves stress/tension, purifies and cleanses, rehydrates, cools, antidepressant, good on dry skin, considered "queen of flowers," most expensive, least toxic of all essences.
Rosemary (herb):	Antiseptic, universal aid, toning, helps memory loss, very stimulating, analgesic, invigorating, reduces muscle soreness.
Sage (herb):	Stimulant, astringent, antiseptic, uplifting, restores energy of whole system, toning.
Sandalwood (wood):	Antiseptic, astringent, sedative, toning, antidepressant, reduces nervous tension, soothing, good for acne.
Spearmint (herb):	Stimulant, similar to camphor, cooling then heating, antiseptic, soothes redness, invigorating.
Tea tree (wood):	Antibacterial/fungicidal/virucidal, sudorific, great for acne, powerful immune stimulant, energizes.
Thyme (herb):	Antiseptic, reduces fatigue, germicidal, nonirritating. (Caution: must be diluted.)

Wintergreen (leaves):	Antiseptic, analgesic, relieves sore muscles and joints. (Caution: must be diluted.)
Ylang ylang (flower):	Sedative, calms nerves, antidepressant, decongestive, relaxing, one of most pleasant to use, good on oily skin, euphoric. (Caution: must be diluted.)

Calming	Stimulating	Astringent	Moisturizing	Antistress Antidepressant	Antiinflammatory	Antibacterial Antiacne Oil	Analgesic
Melissa	Rosemary	Rosemary	Orange	Chamomile	Chamomile	Tea Tree	Lavender
Rose	Camphor	Birch	Rose	Geranium	Lavender	Bergamot	Chamomile
Geranium	Thyme	Cedarwood	Chamomile	Lavender	Geranium	Cedarwood	Camphor
Lavender	Clove	Cypress	Neroli	Sandalwood	Jasmine	Lemon	Clove
Clary Sage	Cinnamon	Frankincense	Patchouli	Ylang Ylang	Neroli	Lemongrass	Eucalyptus
Chamomile	Eucalyptus	Grapefruit		Basil		Myrrh	Oregano
Jasmine	Pine	Juniper		Melissa		Peppermint	Peppermint
Eucalyptus	Spearmint	Myrrh		Neroli		Thyme	Rosemary
Ylang Ylang	Peppermint	Sandalwood		Sage		Ylang Ylang	Wintergreen
Frankincense	Oregano	Sage		Sandalwood			
Camphor							

*All are antiseptic to some degree

Combinations and How to Use Them

The previous list represents only a small group of the most common. You will see a lot of overlap. Oils may be used singly or in combination with others. Normally all oils will be diluted into a carrier oil. This carrier oil is normally a vegetable oil and is generally chosen in consideration of the skin condition. The essential oils are put into the carrier oil. The typical safe formula ratio is 2 percent essential oil to the carrier oil. This means about 20–25 drops per 2 ounces of carrier oil. This formula will vary according to the application. For massage use 25 drops per 2 ounces carrier oil; 2 ounces per person is plenty. For a bath use 10–30 drops or 10 drops per tablespoon carrier oil if put in bath as combination. For an infusion use 7–10 drops per quart of water. (Room diffusers are sold by various companies specializing in aroma essences.) For compresses use 2–3 drops per 6 inches on wet gauze or linen square.

CAUTION: THESE ARE GENERAL FORMULAS. PLEASE CONSULT YOUR SUPPLIER FOR SPECIFIC RECIPES AND FORMULAS DUE TO POTENTIAL TOXICITY.

CARRIER OILS

Carrier oils should be vegetable based. Some good oil suggestions follow:

DRY SKIN	COMBINATION	OILY
Sweet Almond Oil	Corn Oil	Grapeseed Oil
Olive Oil	Jojoba Oil	Hazelnut Oil
Palm Kernel Oil	Sesame Oil	Sunflower Oil

SOME SUGGESTED COMBINATIONS

Normally essential oils work well by themselves or in combinations of three to five. Too many added together may dilute the effects. The following combinations will contain only three for simplicity. Again, depending on your goals, consult your supplier for specific recipes.

FACE

Combination skin:	Geranium, Neroli, Ylang Ylang
Acne:	Bergamot, Chamomile, Tea Tree
Dry skin:	Rose, Lavender, Chamomile
Oily skin:	Clary Sage, Lavender, Camphor,
Couperose:	Cypress, Patchouli, Chamomile
Sensitive skin:	Rose, Chamomile, Neroli
Mature skin:	Frankincense, Neroli, Rose

BODY

Overall Well-being:	Geranium, Melissa, Lavender
Relaxing:	Lavender, Ylang Ylang, Melissa
Stress Reduction:	Lavender, Chamomile, Ylang Ylang
Muscle Relief:	Pine, Rosemary, Juniper
Invigorating:	Lavender, Rosemary, Thyme
Circulation:	Grapefruit, Lemon, Geranium
Cellulite:	Fennel, Rosemary, Lavender
Men's Bath:	Sandalwood, Pine, Lemon
Relaxation Bath:	Rose, Lavender, Jasmine
Stimulating Bath:	Peppermint, Pine, Lavender
Foot Bath:	Tea Tree, Rosemary, Sage

> COMBINATIONS BASED ON FRAGRANCE ONLY
>
> Floral: Rose, Jasmine
> Oriental: Ylang Ylang, Jasmine, Neroli, Camphor
> Spicy: Clove, Cinnamon
> Woodsy: Sandalwood, Pine, Cypress, Camphor
> Fruity: Lemon, Grapefruit, Orange

The combinations listed may not suit you or any given client. It's always wise at the beginning of the treatment in the spa to ask the client if the fragrance is pleasing. If it is irritating, it must be changed. Innumerable combinations will be pleasant to the client and still accomplish your goals. As you have seen, all essential oils are antiseptic to one degree or another so the versatility is obvious. There are many other overlapping oils from which you may choose. And the above list is not extensive. This is why it's so important to attend classes, visit with many manufacturers, and learn more about oils.

· ·

SPA POINT

Combinations should be selected with the client's pleasure in mind. If the scent is unpleasant, a great deal of the value of the treatment is lost. Be sure to ask the client.

· ·

Contraindications

As has been stated over and over again, aromatherapy is wonderful, but you must take caution. Some essential oils are highly toxic if used in too strong a concentration or for too long. Oils can have a pleasing effect or make the client nauseous. The following lists some of the contraindications to treatment.

- Pregnancy.
- Any systemic disease such as cancer or diabetes. Obtain physician's release.
- Open wounds, areas of infection or inflammation.
- Allergic reactions and skin rashes.
- Telangiectasia (couperose, varicose veins).
- High/low blood pressure.
- Whenever in doubt, don't!

THE TREATMENT AND AFTER

Room diffusers are great to turn on a few minutes before the client arrives, but then turn them off. Many therapists become so used to the scent that they don't realize how strong it is and the client can become very uncomfortable, develop a headache, or become nauseated. Keep the diffusers under control.

Typically, the aromatherapy treatment itself is incorporated into the massage. Therefore, the essential oils are chosen, added to the carrier oil if not already blended, and then the massage is performed. If you are unsure of combining oils, it may be more appropriate for you to use preblended ones.

After the treatment, the client should be given water and allowed a little time to rebalance and normalize before leaving the room. The client may be very thirsty, have to urinate often, and may be sleepy. This is normal. Advise client to stay out of the sun, saunas, baths, or any heating-up situation for 5 hours. Even after that time, the client should avoid the sun because essential oils are often photosensitive and can potentially cause splotchiness of the skin. Due to the natural detoxifying that will normally take place, alcohol should not be consumed, and drinking lots of water is recommended for the next 24 hours.

Synopsis

Aromatherapy is a wonderful and very active science in the professional's repertoire of treatment capabilities. Aromatherapy is a vital part of all beauty and well-being concepts now and well into the future. The great part is that it's all natural and has already stood the test of time. We are just now unlocking the treasure chest of treatment modalities that have been around for four thousand or more years. From frankincense and myrrh in Christ's day to rose oil in ours, the joy and satisfaction from nature's treasure is yours to explore and expand.

Review

1. Who is considered to have developed the art of aromatherapy and coined the word?

2. How long has the use of natural plants been around? Give an example from the Bible.

3. What are the "king" and "queen" of flowers and why?

4. What combination has been recommended for combination skin?

5. What are two of the contraindications of aromatherapy?

6. Why is aromatherapy important in day spa treatments?

CHAPTER 7
Client Preparation and Room Setup

OVERVIEW

Body work requires greater diligence in client care than a facial treatment. For the esthetician expanding into body treatment, it's vital to understand that you are now treating a much larger area than just the face. Where there has been significance in charting and knowing contraindications of treatment for the face, the same is true in a different and larger capacity on the body. In facial treatments we are primarily concerned with contraindications that might cause a reaction to the products and procedures done on the face. When it comes to body treatments allergic reactions may occur, but we are more concerned with overall health and circulatory issues that may determine the safety of a particular body treatment. This is not to scare the esthetician, but the technician needs to make certain adjustments in concepts.

For the massage therapist accustomed only to performing massage, there will be an entirely new world of treatment understanding and client relations. For the progressive massage therapist, this will be a joy and challenge to growth. For the massage therapist who doesn't particularly believe in the value of products, the learning may come harder. For the cosmetologist or other beauty professional, this opens up an entirely new scope of growth and learning. Some thought will have to be given to how to grow into this field, but the client handling will be a large and critical aspect of success in day spa work. That is why an entire chapter is being devoted to client preparation.

BASIC CLIENT PREPARATION

There are many important basic concepts involved in handling clients for body work. The technician needs to expand his or her scope of skin and wellness consciousness. While some estheticians are still just trying to get clients to purchase a cleanser, freshener, and moisturizer the idea of trying to get the client to think of body treatments and products is like telling the average person that he will take a trip to the moon. The client must be educated into day spa body treatments. A small minority of clients travel to destination spas and like body treatments so much that they will ask for them on their own, but the vast majority must be educated and encouraged to take treatments. How this takes place will be covered more fully in *Day Spa Operations*.

Another aspect of body treatment that will need to be worked through with the client is the idea of taking clothes off and being worked on "in the buff" by a technician. Most people feel that their body is not good enough to be seen by anyone. First of all, with the possible exception of a Scotch hose or other similar treatment, the only part of the body seen by the technician at any one time is the part being worked on. This seems obvious to the technician but the client must be educated to understand this so that taking clothes off isn't a hindrance to growth into the wonderful world of body care. Caution and attention to proper draping will resolve the issue once the client has been in for a treatment, but initially shyness is an obstacle that must be handled.

Both of these major obstacles are not difficult and most often can be handled well from the outset by having a good quality consultation chart.

The Consultation Chart

If your consultation chart is extensive enough to handle all areas of your day spa, it can be filled out the first time a client comes in for any service. The client should be asked to arrive 10–15 minutes early on the first visit to allow time for filling out the chart. This is the same procedure physicians use so it shouldn't receive much, if any, resistance from the client. The information contained in the chart will allow the technician to grow the client—even if a client came in for nail care, the information should be helpful to graduate that client into spa manicures and pedicures as well as into other full-body treatments. One of the best types of consultation charts available is the kind printed on manilla folders, the outside having information for the client to fill out and the inside set aside for the technicians.

BASIC QUESTIONS ON CHART FROM A CLIENT STANDPOINT

You must have an area for the client to fill out name; address; phone number; occupation; date of birth (hopefully the client will answer this one as it's helpful for promotions, etc.); and physicians' names, addresses, and phone numbers (family physician and dermatologist).

There needs to be an area listing as many common diseases and disorders as possible for the client to check off. Important issues for body treatment are allergies, birth control pills, blood disorders (high and low blood pressure, phlebitis, varicose veins, diabetes, etc.), cancer, any systemic disease, hypo- or hyperthyroid, inflammation, infection, medications (internal as well as topical), pacemaker, pregnancy, rashes (local or systemic), recent surgeries, and any other questionable condition. Having this information will eliminate the possibility of treatment without first receiving a physician's release. This is for your safety as well as the client's safety.

You should know basically what products the client uses on the face as well as the body. These may be listed so that the client checks a box or you may prefer to write them down as you discuss skin care with the client. When beginning to do body treatments, it's important to know what kinds of products the client uses at home as well as products the client may be interested in. (Figure 7-1)

There should also be an area to discern lifestyle habits. Does this person exercise regularly? Is the person active and health oriented or sedentary and generally not concerned? It's good to inquire about areas of interest in body treatments, past experiences, and so forth. A favorite question to

CLIENT CONSULTATION FORM

Name _____

Address _____

City _____ State _____ Zip _____

Home # _____ Business # _____

Fax # _____ Car # _____

Occupation _____

Date of Birth _____

Marital Status _____ Spouse's Name _____

Family Physician _____ Phone # _____

Dermatologist _____ Phone # _____

Last Seen: ○ Physician   ○ Dermatologist   ○ Other _____

Reason for Last Doctor's Visit: _____ Date _____

MEDICAL HISTORY

Check Box Where Applicable / Fill In With Details:

○ Accutane	○ Acne
○ Allergies _____	○ Arthritis
○ Artificial Implants	○ Asthma
○ Birth Control _____	○ Blood Disorder
○ Blood Thinner	○ Cancer _____
○ Claustrophobia	○ Contact Lens
○ Depression	○ Diabetic
○ Distended Capillaries	○ Eczema
○ Epilepsy	○ Fever Blisters
○ Heart Condition	○ Hepatitis
○ High Blood Pressure	○ HIV
○ Hyper/Hypo Pigmentation	○ Hyper/Hypo Thyroid
○ Insomnia	○ Lupus
○ Medication _____	○ Metal Plates or Pins
○ Nail Disorders	○ Pacemaker
○ Phlebitis	○ Plastic Surgery _____
○ Pregnant	○ Psoriasis
○ Retin-A®	○ Scleroderma
○ Seborrhea	○ Sensitivites
○ Skin Cancer _____	○ Surgeries _____
○ Underweight/Overweight	○ Vitamins
○ Other: _____	

PERSONAL SKIN CARE HISTORY

Please Check Current Products You Use:

○ Eye Make-Up Remover	○ Cleansing Cream/Lotion	○ Facial Soap
○ Skin Freshener (Toner, Astringent)	○ Day Cream	○ Night Cream
○ Eye Cream	○ Neck Cream	○ Mask
○ Facial Scrub	○ Exfoliants	○ Body Soap
○ Body Lotion/Cream	○ Body Scrub	○ Hand Cream
○ Sunscreen # _____	○ Other: _____	

FIGURE 7-1 *The client consultation form should ask about the client's medical and personal skin care history, as well as record the client's address and phone numbers.*

ask is how the client thinks of his or her own body condition and what areas he/she would like to improve. (Figure 7-2)

BASIC ANALYSIS AND CONCERNS ON CHART FROM TECHNICIAN STANDPOINT

If a client has shown interest in body treatments, don't be surprised if that person isn't quite honest with the health history. When doing certain treatments, such as a 30-minute hydrotherapy tub treatment, you should ask about contraindications again. You may also want to include a disclaimer

PERSONAL EVALUATION QUESTIONNAIRE

PLEASE REPLY IN DETAIL TO THE FOLLOWING QUESTIONS:

1. How did you hear about our salon? _____

2. What is your major reason for being here today? _____

3. What skin type and/or problems do you feel you have? _____

4. Have you ever had a facial treatment before? If yes, where and when? Was it a beneficial experience? _____

5. Have you ever had a reaction to a cosmetic or skin care product? Please describe. _____

6. Have you ever had a body/bust treatment? _____

7. Where do you purchase most of your face and body care products? _____

8. How much time do you spend on your daily skin care/make-up routine? _____

9. How do you feel about your body and skin conditions? What would you like to improve? _____

10. Do you tend to tan or burn? _____

11. Do you smoke? _____

12. Do you exercise? How much? _____

13. How much sleep do you get per night? _____

14. How much do you drink of the following:

	Little	Moderate	Heavy
Water	O	O	O
Coffee	O	O	O
Tea	O	O	O
Alcohol	O	O	O
Soft Drinks	O	O	O

15. Would you like to be on our mailing list for promotions and classes? _____

16. Are you interested in long or short term salon treatment? _____

17. Are you pleased with your current products? _____

18. Have you ever been waxed with depilatory wax before? _____

SALON POLICIES

I understand fully and agree to comply with all the salon policies listed below:

1. We do not wax anyone on Accutane, Retin-A®, or other medications/products that exfoliate or thin the skin. We do not wax anyone undergoing chemotherapy or radiation treatments.
2. We will not treat clients with questionable medical conditions such as herpes simplex (cold sores, fever blisters), open wounds or sores, healing incisions, infectious dieases, etc. We do not massage clients undergoing cancer, diabetic, or systemic treatments or any other specific contra-indications to body treatments.
3. We require a minimum of 24 hours advance cancellation notice. Any client giving less will be charged that full fee of service reserved.
4. I understand that the services received here are not a substitute for medical care and any information provided by the esthetician is for educational purposes only.
5. All information received by the client on this chart is completely private and confidential.
6. We do not give cash refunds.
7. Defective products must be returned within 10 days of purchase to recieve credit.

_____   _____
Date   Signature

FIGURE 7-2 *Use the client consultation form as a way to familiarize yourself with your client. Ask questions that will help you assess the best kind of treatment for the client.*

on the chart listing some conditions that won't be treated without a release from the client's doctor. Some people just don't tell the truth, particularly about medications.

As stated before, the technician must discuss treatments in terms of removing clothes and being nude. The clients must feel confident about their modesty being protected, particularly at first. Confidence and less modesty will naturally result with experience, but initially it can be a large obstacle to obtaining treatments.

TECHNICAL ANALYSIS

PLEASE REPLY IN DETAIL TO THE FOLLOWING QUESTIONS

SKIN TYPE:
- ○ Acne
- ○ Combination
- ○ Normal
- ○ Alipidic
- ○ Dehydrated
- ○ Oily

SKIN CONDITIONS:
- ○ Aged
- ○ Bruising
- ○ Comedones
- ○ Distended Capillaries
- ○ Fine Lines
- ○ Hyper Pigmentation
- ○ Milia
- ○ Papules
- ○ Sagging Bust Line
- ○ Stretch Marks
- ○ Wrinkles
- ○ Birthmarks
- ○ Cellulite
- ○ Dark Circles
- ○ Excessive Hair
- ○ Flaccid, Sagging
- ○ Hypo Pigmentation
- ○ Moles
- ○ Pustules
- ○ Scars
- ○ Warts
- ○ Other: _____

NAILS:
Type
- ○ Brittle
- ○ Dry
- ○ Damaged
- ○ Normal

Conditions
- ○ Callouses
- ○ Hangnails
- ○ Weak
- ○ Chipped
- ○ Thin
- ○ Other: _____

MASSAGE:
Areas of Stress
- ○ Back
- ○ Hips
- ○ Lumbar
- ○ Shoulders
- ○ Feet (Right/Left)
- ○ Legs
- ○ Neck
- ○ Thoracic

Type of Massage
- ○ Shiatsu
- ○ Swedish

Result
- ○ Headaches
- ○ Sciatic
- ○ Lower Back Pain
- ○ Other: _____

SKIN TEXTURE/COLOR:
- ○ Albino
- ○ Enlarged Pores
- ○ Grayed
- ○ Pale
- ○ Pitting
- ○ Ruddy
- ○ Smooth
- ○ Tanned
- ○ Thin
- ○ Black
- ○ Ethnic
- ○ Olive
- ○ Pink
- ○ Rough
- ○ Shallow
- ○ Sunburned
- ○ Thick
- ○ Other: _____

UPDATE ANALYSIS

Date	Comments

FIGURE 7-3 *Record your analysis of the client on the form.*

The technician should always analyze the skin as the treatments are being performed. This will be particularly helpful in areas the client can't see, such as the back. Any potential skin lesion/cancer should be pointed out and charted (Figure 7-3). The client should be encouraged to see a physician about any questionable lesions or growths. Any open wounds or areas of inflammation should be avoided entirely and charted. Skin and muscle tone should also be considered. Areas of stress or discomfort should be charted along with areas to be avoided. Skin color, texture, and degree of dehydration/scaliness should be a major area of treatment concentration and thus charted.

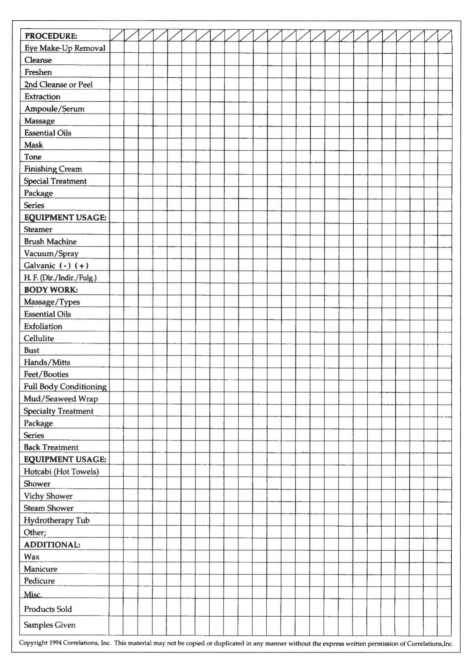

PROCEDURE:																		
Eye Make-Up Removal																		
Cleanse																		
Freshen																		
2nd Cleanse or Peel																		
Extraction																		
Ampoule/Serum																		
Massage																		
Essential Oils																		
Mask																		
Tone																		
Finishing Cream																		
Special Treatment																		
Package																		
Series																		
EQUIPMENT USAGE:																		
Steamer																		
Brush Machine																		
Vacuum/Spray																		
Galvanic (-) (+)																		
H. F. (Dir./Indir./Fulg.)																		
BODY WORK:																		
Massage/Types																		
Essential Oils																		
Exfoliation																		
Cellulite																		
Bust																		
Hands/Mitts																		
Feet/Booties																		
Full Body Conditioning																		
Mud/Seaweed Wrap																		
Specialty Treatment																		
Package																		
Series																		
Back Treatment																		
EQUIPMENT USAGE:																		
Hotcabi (Hot Towels)																		
Shower																		
Vichy Shower																		
Steam Shower																		
Hydrotherapy Tub																		
Other;																		
ADDITIONAL:																		
Wax																		
Manicure																		
Pedicure																		
Misc.																		
Products Sold																		
Samples Given																		

FIGURE 7-4 *Keep track of the equipment used, products sold, and procedures completed on each visit.*

The technician must remember the health issues and contraindications and must consider each one in view of the treatment planned each time. Certain treatments can be performed and others might not be able to be done. Good consciousness of the client will help determine safety here.

The technician must keep great records of treatments given (Figure 7-4), goals to achieve, reasons for series and effects, along with anything unusual on the body that might be cause for concern. And even if the client visits regularly, the technician should remember to ask updated health questions. At a very minimum, the technician should ask if there have been any changes in the health or condition of the client since last seen.

It's important to keep records in the chart of products sold as well as those recommended. Samples given should be recorded for follow-up in a few days.

· ·

SPA POINT

Keeping good consultation charts is not an option, it's a requirement of the professional. Keeping the charts filled out and updated will go far in achieving success in the treatments, home care programs, and in protecting both the client and technician from mistakes.

· ·

WET ROOM VERSUS DRY ROOM

Wet Room

As stated previously, a wet room is a room that has been constructed in such a way that it can get wet without damaging the room. Most wet rooms are completely tiled up to the ceilings and have floor drains. The room must be constructed in such a way that the floor is sloped for quick drainage. The ceiling must be made of waterproof materials. If tiles are used for the floor and walls, which is recommended, the grouting must be mold and mildew resistant. In other words, the room must be constructed to be conducive to being wet all day long. Depending on what is being done, the wet room should be about 9 feet by 12 feet in size. If you plan to include a Scotch hose in the wet room with a tub, you might consider going 10 feet by 14 feet for sufficient room to do both. In addition to room size, all wet rooms should have a shower and hand-held hose to allow for the client to shower as well as for ease of cleanup and to wash down the walls and drain the floor quickly. It's a good idea to have indirect lighting that is waterproof and controlled by a dimmer switch to add to the room ambiance.

TREATMENTS IDEALLY SUITED TO A WET ROOM

- Hydrotherapy tub treatment.

- Vichy shower treatment along with all showering devices.

- Scotch hose treatment.

- Body treatments such as salt glows, mud masks, and seaweed wraps work well in the wet room. Mud is easier to remove in a wet room than in a dry treatment room. This may vary somewhat according to the product.

Overall, any and all body treatments can easily and comfortably be done in the wet room. Conversely, some body treatments may be done in a dry room but are better suited to the wet areas.

RULES OF THE WET ROOM

- The room must be cleaned, sanitized, and dried between each client. The client must enter a wet area feeling that he or she is the first client to ever touch that room.

- Some seaweeds and mud can stain certain types of tiles so be sure to clean the tiles immediately after use to avoid staining. When purchasing tiles, be sure they are water and stain resistant or stain proof.

- The floor must be sloped and fitted with drainage systems that drain a floor quickly.

- Glass objects including drinking glasses and bowls should never be used in a wet room.

Dry Room

This is a massage or treatment room, normally not tiled or drained for water. A dry room is often more relaxing and conducive to massage and some types of treatments. It's valuable to have a shower attached or nearby to facilitate product removal. But the room itself will be much quieter without the tile and it gives a more soothing ambiance to the client. The typical dry room size is about 8 feet by 10 feet. It can actually be a little smaller, but smaller than this will often give a closed in, claustrophobic sensation to the client. It's good to have a sink in the room for preparing and washing out treatment bowls and the like. If a sink is not possible, the technician needs to have a water source nearby. Most facilities considering body treatments tend to ignore the value of plumbing for a sink in the treatment rooms because they think of the room strictly for massage. Although it is not absolutely necessary, it is still a good idea to have a sink if for no other reason than to be able to wash hands in front of the client or to warm the massage oil. Again, the sink must be kept clean, sanitized, and dried between clients. The floor covering should be easy to keep up. Some states prohibit carpet and in some senses tile is better. However, tile is hard on the technician's feet. If using a floor covering such as carpet, be sure it's vacuumed after treatments.

TREATMENTS IDEALLY SUITED TO A DRY ROOM

- Massage.

- Salt or body polishes if a shower is nearby.

- Seaweed wraps.

- All spot treatments.

Remember, it isn't that all treatments, including mud, can't be done in a dry room, but it's easier and more efficient to do certain messy or difficult to remove treatments in a wet area as opposed to a dry area.

RULES OF THE DRY ROOM

- The floor covering should be something easy to clean up, sweep, dust, or vacuum after removal of treatments such as exfoliants and salts.

- Do not use any glass objects that can fall and break. It's difficult to be sure all pieces of glass are completely picked up.

- Indirect lighting on dimmer switches is important. The room should also be wired for music.

- A clean, crisp bed setup should be done after each client, even if another client isn't due soon. The look of a room already set up makes the day spa look professional and becomes inviting to a client on tour.

• •

SPA POINT

Wet rooms with tiling all around and good floor drainage are more conducive to the difficult, messy, or hard to remove treatments such as mud. Cleaning, sanitizing, and drying the wet room between clients is imperative!

• •

ROOM AMBIANCE

The ambiance or mood of the rooms is important. Remember, you're dealing with Americans who still tend to be a little shy about body treatments. If the rooms are pristine, clean, and welcoming, the client's reluctance is reduced and your ability to make progress in body treatment services is greatly heightened.

The room must be pristine and immaculately clean, sanitized, dry. Sheets and towels must be clean, fresh, and without oil stains or odors. There are a number of products on the market available to remove the rancid smell and stain from oils. The bed must be made up between clients and look fresh, as if nobody had ever been on those sheets before. Replace old sheets and towels when necessary to preserve this image. All implements and surfaces must be cleaned and disinfected between clients.

Oil and other product containers must also be clean and pleasant looking. Do not allow massage oil bottles to look old, dirty, or rancid. Purchase new bottles when necessary to maintain a very clean, fresh look. All products should be displayed well. This is a form of indirect selling and a good display will help market both your retail products and services.

The room colors, lighting, and mood should be very inviting and relaxing, ideally to both men and women if you have a mixed clientele. Pink walls might be fine for a woman and brown great for a man, but either would be disaster for a mixed clientele. Subtle taupes, beiges, or greys are more conducive to men and women alike. Keep both sexes in mind when choosing lighting. The lighting should be subdued and controlled by a dimmer switch so that it can be raised or lowered during consultation and treatment times.

Professional attire for the technician is a must. The clothing or uniform should be fresh, clean, and dry. Sometimes it is necessary to change clothes several times a day due to water splashing from hydrotherapy equipment.

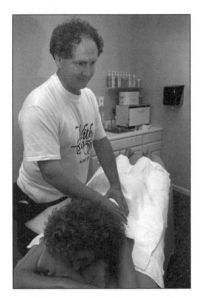

FIGURE 7-5 *The technician must be in comfortable but professional attire.*

A dirty or stained lab coat can kill your business. Create some type of uniform (Figure 7-5). Street clothes are not appropriate. Whatever uniform you decide on, be sure it looks professional. This will go a long way in relieving shyness on the part of the client as well portraying your professionalism and taking the "person" out of the impression.

It's a good idea to have a clock on the wall that the technician can watch to maintain timeliness and promptness without being too obvious to the client. And music is a great addition to the room. It is better if done through a speaker system than with a jam box and tapes piled up on the counter. If not feasible, be sure the tapes are kept in a container and the jam box clean. Music of choice should be relaxing and quiet, such as Yanni, Windham Hill, etc.

• •

SPA POINT

The ambiance of the room makes a large impact on the client. A welcoming, relaxing, warm room will entice and calm a client before a treatment even begins. Cleanliness is not only next to Godliness, it's tantamount to success or failure. An unclean room will scare off a potential client without you even realizing it.

• •

Bed Setup

The setup of the bed depends heavily on what types of treatments are being done. In any case, the bed must be made comfortable and warm. The bed may be set up differently in a dry room versus a wet room. In addition to sheets, towels, and blankets, body treatments will now utilize Mylar foil or plastic for wrapping purposes. In some cases gauze, muslin, or linen sheets will also be used with treatments for wrapping or covering the client.

FOIL

This isn't kitchen aluminum foil. The Mylar foil is ideally suited to close wrapping and is normally used for treatments where you want more heat generated. Think of foil for cooking to help you remember when you want to use it. Foil is often used for cellulite treatments and seaweed treatments when perspiration and body warmth is desired.

Some people suggest using space blankets and camping blankets that you can purchase in a sporting goods store. These will work, but there may be questionable success in washing and properly disinfecting the blanket. The advantage of a space blanket is the reusability, but it's quite dangerous if you are not absolutely certain of the disinfection. It is recommended to use disposable Mylar foil sheets and to discard after each client. When doing a full-body treatment, the size of the foil should be about 6 feet by 6 feet. Then, in partial treatments, the size of the foil should be cut oversize to completely envelop the area being treated. For example, the foil size for a cellulite treatment should be about 4 feet by 6 feet to wrap both legs. Obviously the size of the foil depends somewhat on the size of the body.

PLASTIC

This also isn't kitchen-version wrap. The texture should be the thickness of tall kitchen garbage bags. Plastic normally comes in a roll and can be cut to size. Sizes for plastic will be the same as foil. Once again, some technicians like to use shower curtain liners and wash after use. If this is your choice, be aware that disinfection is again difficult. Also if you do use shower curtain liners, be sure to cut off the area where the holes are. It is recommended to use disposable plastic sheets.

Wet Room Bed Setup

The bed itself should be waterproof or water resistant. This means purchasing a special wet room table or using a metal or plastic table with some kind of waterproof covering. Many beginning spas use plastic tables with foam mattresses used in the pool or at the ocean. Some wet rooms use tile tables. Whatever is used, be sure it is covered with something comfortable for the client to lay on. Then this is covered with foil or plastic, depending on the treatment being done. If only a massage is being done without any water, the bed can be set up as in a dry room.

A towel should cover the headrest part of the foam mattress or be rolled up comfortably under the client's head to elevate it slightly. Other towels may be needed under the small of the back or under the knees for added comfort. These towels will get wet and should be removed after the wet portion of treatment. If a massage is to follow a wet treatment in the same room, the client should be asked to get up and wait in a chair while the bed is prepared again. This time the bed should be dry, with new sheets and towels. Again a bolster or towels may be placed under the head, back, and knees.

Dry towels should always be put on the floor as a bath mat for the client to step on.

Dry Room Bed Setup

The setup may depend on the treatment or treatments being performed. But as a rule, the bed will first be covered with an electric bed warmer (not electric blanket for you should not lie on an electric blanket, whereas bed warmers are designed for people to lie on), then a light blanket, sheet, then bath towel. At this point the choice of foil or plastic will depend on the treatment. Sometimes both will be put down if the treatment is being layered. For example, when doing a salt glow and a seaweed body wrap, the foil will be put over the towel and then the plastic will be put over the foil. After the salt glow is completed, the plastic will be rolled out from under the client, leaving the client lying on the foil.

After the client has been wrapped in foil or plastic, the bed warmer is turned off, the client is further wrapped in the sheet and blanket. A bolster or towels may then be placed under the head, back, and knees for added comfort.

After the treatment wrap has been completed, normally after about 15–30 minutes, the blanket and sheet are opened. The client's foil or plastic is loosened and then the client is helped to a standing position and allowed to enter the shower with the foil or plastic still wrapped around. The client is instructed to remove and just drop the foil/plastic, to shower off the mud or seaweed or whatever product is on the skin. While the client is showering the bed is freshened and a new cover bath towel or preferably bath sheet is readied for covering the client. The client is given a fresh dry towel with which to dry off, then is robed and escorted back to the bed to complete the treatment. The bed warmer should have been turned on again to help ensure that the client doesn't get chilled.

• •

SPA POINT

Whether working in a wet or dry room, proper draping and careful covering of the client is imperative. Fresh clean towels should be used after every exposure to water. Do not make the client use the same towel to dry off after a shower, tub, etc. Clients feel more luxurious if bath sheets are used to cover them than just bath towels. Bath sheets give a rich aura and cover the client better than bath towels.

• •

Work Area Setup

Tools and supplies must be kept immaculately clean and sanitized. The work area should be neat and inviting to the client, never crowded or messy. Bottles must be clean and pleasant looking. Be sure the products to be used on the client are lined up on a towel on the counter to make a welcoming effect. Clutter is an absolute no-no!

SUPPLIES NEEDED

1. Plastic mixing bowls and metal mixing bowls. It is preferable not to mix or dispense muds in metal containers. On the other hand, white plastic sometimes stains with seaweed so metal is sometimes better for seaweeds. Otherwise, wash and disinfect immediately to avoid staining as much as possible. Some of the blue plastic containers at the grocery store will work well and stain little. Never use glass containers or implements, particularly in a wet area. The only glass allowed would be the essential oil bottles that must be packaged in glass. But be cautious and never have them near the tub or tables where they might slip, break, and splinter.

2. Metal and wooden whisks and large plastic spoons for mixing seaweed powders and other products.

3. Measuring cups for additives.

4. Disinfectant for spraying surfaces and hands, wet sanitizer containing disinfectant for implements, and dry storage container for implements and sponges after disinfection. Check into your state and federal requirements for disinfectants.

5. Sponges, shammies, brushes, loofah mitts, etc. All supplies that are needed to perform various exfoliation, rinsing, and washing capabilities. Be sure these are all implements that can be disinfected.

Towels

You will use many towels per treatment. For every trip to the shower or water source, you will need a bath towel or bath sheet. You will need two bath towels for bath mats at the work table as well as for the tub or shower. Then you will need two to three bath sheets for covering the client during treatment depending on the number of treatments combined. You may need extra towels for bolsters under the head, back, knees. You will use a minimum of five towels per water treatment. Remember, after any water treatment the client will return to the bed for lotion application. This will require a fresh towel on the bed and to cover the client.

Sheets

Normally only one or two sheets are used per treatment. If the first sheet is well covered with toweling, it may not be necessary to use a second sheet. But if the sheet is the primary covering tool, then two to three sheets will be needed. When using the wet room for a wet treatment such as the Vichy shower and then for massage, two to three sheets will be necessary.

A final note on sheets, towels, and supplies—be sure they are in good shape. When they get old and thin, it is advisable to replace them. Since the day spa is a spin-off from the destination spa, luxurious sheets and towels are more success oriented. Purchasing high-quality sheets and towels may cost more, but they will certainly last longer and give a much better impression.

· ·

SPA POINT

The image a client of day spas requires is that of high quality and luxury. The cleanliness and presentation of towels, sheets, bed setup, and rooms are a critical part of the success of the operation. The operative words are quality *and pro-fessionalism.*

· ·

Synopsis

This chapter is entirely concerned with issues that may seem unimportant but that can make or break the business. Americans are still shy about taking their clothes off. If the client is assured by the appearance and professionalism that their modesty will be protected and that the treatment is hygienically safe, then the business will prosper. If the client feels that the work rooms and areas are unsanitary, the business will die without you even knowing what happened. Disinfection and sanitation are critical. Employees must also understand that wet areas must be cleaned, sanitized, and dried after each client and that if there isn't an assistant for that job, then the cleanup is a natural part of the client treatment. Sheets and towels must also be fresh, clean, and inviting looking; old, stained, thin towels are not appropriate for a successful day spa operation.

Review

1. Is shyness a consideration when introducing clients to body treatments?

2. What concerns make body work different from facial work?

3. How should the issue of removing clothes and being "in the buff" be handled?

4. What is the difference between a wet and dry room?

5. Should anything made of glass be allowed in a treatment area? Why?

6. What is the difference between an electric blanket and bed warmer in treatments?

7. Why are bath sheets preferable to bath towels in some cases?

CHAPTER 8
Body Treatments and Treatment Development _____

OVERVIEW

This is an exciting chapter because we will begin to develop the day spa treatment program. In subsequent chapters we'll highlight some of the critical treatment topics such as exfoliants, mud, and seaweed. In order to better understand the ingredients, it's useful to understand the development of treatments first. As with anything, there are a myriad of treatment capabilities for the day spa and variations may occur within one product line that don't in another. In keeping with a simple day spa concept, we will not dwell on specific product line applications. Marketing and menu development will be covered in detail in *Day Spa Operations*.

In this chapter we will look at overall goals and treatments to suit those goals, general contraindications, and scheduling treatments with and without hydrotherapy. It can be a little difficult to develop a full program without knowing the specifics of an individual day spa. However, general principles will normally work for all sizes and market strata.

BODY TREATMENT CONCEPTS

Why are body treatments important? Why is a day spa based on body treatment? Why should we bother selling combinations of treatments? These are only a few of the questions you need to ask yourself when going into the day spa business. You must have a clear-cut target in order to make it work.

As has been discussed in previous chapters, the American consumer is still learning how to take care of the face, much less consider the body. Estheticians and massage therapists have little experience themselves in body work with products and treatments, which can make passing the idea on to the client more difficult. Even with the advent of all the destination spas, spa books, and spa travel agencies there is still a feeling of luxury and vacation about body care. The ultimate concept you must address with your client is:

> BODY CARE IS A NECESSITY FOR HEALTH, WELL-BEING, AND YOUTHFUL APPEARANCE. IT IS NOT JUST A LUXURY TO BE ENJOYED FROM TIME TO TIME. YOUR BODY IS THE ONLY ONE YOU'LL EVER GET SO IT'S IMPORTANT TO MAKE THE MOST OF IT NOW!

To achieve this, the technician must believe the following:

1. Body care really is important and valuable.

2. Body treatments really do work.

3. Hydrotherapy really is therapy for well-being all by itself.

4. Hydrotherapy in conjunction with other product-based treatment will further enhance the benefits of either alone.

5. There is a difference in professional products and treatments from over-the-counter body products.

6. With consistent treatment, the person can feel and look better.

7. Although there is no cure for cellulite, a proper all-around program really can help reduce and control cellulite buildup.

8. Body care treatments are worth the investment in time, money, and energy.

9. There is more than just money to be made in body care. There is great personal satisfaction in helping a client be the best that he/she can be.

10. Body care is the wave of the future for the complete skin care professional.

If you are going into this just to make money and you're hassled by the learning curve or the investment, then body care is not for you. For the massage therapist who tends to think of massage only, the learning curve to product and treatment is sometimes difficult, but it is absolutely necessary if you want to succeed.

On the other hand, if body care is an exciting new field of study and you're ready to go, then your day spa has a great chance of success. But remember, it won't take off overnight. Now let's move into the treatment goals.

. . . .

SPA POINT

The most important factor for success in the day spa business is to really believe in the value of body treatments. In most cases this will necessitate the technician's personal experience in giving and receiving treatments. You can't sell what you don't know. You must know firsthand what it's all about!

. . . .

OVERALL TREATMENT GOALS

Body care involves so many things, from hydrotherapy to mud, to seaweed, milk baths, bath salts, lotions and potions, creams and things. What is it all about and how does it work?

TREATMENT GOALS FOR THE CLIENT
- **Relaxation**
- **Skin texture and condition improvement**
- **General wellness enhancement, body invigoration**
- **Relief for stressed, sore, achy muscles**
- **Target and improve specific areas like cellulite, back, or bust**

To accomplish these goals, the following three major categories should fit most treatment concepts.

Exfoliation

Exfoliation is the process whereby the skin is rubbed, polished, or scrubbed or enzymes are used on it to remove dead skin cells, rancid oils, dirt, and debris. There is no question about the effect of life, pollution, and environment on the skin. The life cycle of skin naturally causes dead cells, and with oils and environmental buildup the skin can lose some of its vivacity, tone, and polish. The exfoliation process removes dead cells to bring a more vibrant skin to the surface. The exfoliation also allows the skin to more readily accept moisturizers, nutrients, and treatments designed to improve skin texture or inner skin function. The greatest product in the world is inhibited by an overaccumulation of dead skin. So all the exfoliation goals are designed to improve surface skin texture and prepare the skin for nutrients.

Full-Body Care

Full-body care means exactly that, treatments and products designed to help the entire body. This normally doesn't include the face because of the vast field of technology developed for the face alone. However, they should go hand in hand and preferably be treated together on an ongoing basis. The body is mirrored in the face so both are important. Full-body care in the sense we deal with is not meant to cure disease or disorder but to improve on a basically healthy person. Full-body care is wellness oriented. In other words, it is preventative rather than curative. The work done in day spa treatments may actually relieve a health condition, but that must be an indirect result of the beauty and wellness treatments and never the verbal or actual goal of the technician. No beauty professional or massage therapist is licensed to cure anything. It is very easy to fall into the trap of trying to cure because many of the treatments and products used are, in fact, natural, homeopathic cures, and that's fine but not from a direct healing approach. As a result, the full-body care we are concerned with may be divided into two thoughts.

SKIN CONDITIONING
The skin of the body has texture just as the face does. Body care treatments may be targeted to improve skin texture, color, tone, suppleness, softness, and elasticity.

DETOXIFICATION

A difficult word to express the goal of helping the body to function on its own better. When the circulation and metabolism are stimulated, the body's own processing improves. This in turn improves the elimination process, helping the body to rid itself of wastes and toxins. In other words, this helps the body to detoxify itself. This improved metabolism will help not only the nutritional side of metabolism but also the elimination side. The end result is normally a more energetic, vivacious, active individual who feels more well. We often use the words *detox* or *detoxification* to explain products and treatments that facilitate the body's own natural elimination process.

Spot Treatment

Spot treatment means to work on a portion of the body. Common spot treatments include back, cellulite, bust, hands and arms, feet and calves, or specific stressed areas. The goal in spot treatment normally includes both conditioning of the skin and improvement in metabolism, thus detoxifying and providing nutrition. Spot treatments concentrate on a specific part of the body and may or may not be included in a full-body program. Day spas will offer spot treatments alone very effectively and in conjunction with other full-body concepts very profitably.

Does spot treatment indicate lesser effectiveness than a full-body treatment? No, absolutely not. There will be situations in which one can be quite aggressive on a small area where the full body would be too much. Spot treatment can also provide activity in a more concentrated fashion on that part alone. Combining spot treatments with full-body treatments can be complicated but also exciting. Marketing and combining treatments will be dealt with in more detail in *Day Spa Operations*.

. . . .

SPA POINT

The overall goals are really quite simple when broken down. Body treatments are a process of exfoliation, then treatment for skin conditioning or detoxification on the full body or in spot treatments. Treatments, product ingredients, concepts, and home care all fit into this simply defined treatment goal system.

. . . .

Contraindications

This is a very difficult area for the novice because the contraindications for this treatment and that treatment and then another treatment can be so pervasive that the technician is liable to feel that nobody can be treated. This is not true. Although the conservative answer to contraindications is quite extensive, the bottom line is to consult in detail with the client, obtain a physician's consent and guidance where needed, and proceed very slowly and conservatively in any case where there may be health risks or questions. When we say that high and low blood pressure are contraindications for body treatment, that could potentially eliminate a large part of your client base. Yes, it can be a serious contraindication, but it may also be just a guideline to watch the client carefully.

From a textbook standpoint, you must understand that in body work there are more contraindications to treatment than in facials just by the nature of the size of the area being treated. With extensive experience you'll learn to adjust your treatments, water temperatures, and goals according to the contraindications without necessarily turning away a client. But the beginner is much wiser to adhere strictly to contraindications until the knowledge, experience, and confidence level reach the point where you know exactly what, where, how, and when. And even so, there may be times when the unexpected happens. This is not to scare you but to make you cognizant of the importance of care and proper consultation and charting. Major contraindications are also more important when combining treatment with hydrotherapy or when combining a couple of spot treatments with full-body treatment and then adding hydrotherapy. When in doubt, lesser is better.

> **WHEN IN DOUBT ABOUT WHETHER IT'S OKAY TO TREAT A CLIENT, REDUCE THE TREATMENT TIME, LOWER THE HOT WATER LEVELS, USE LESS OF THE ESSENTIAL OILS AND ACTIVE INGREDIENTS, AND COMBINE FEWER TREATMENTS AND MODALITIES. START SLOWLY AND SIMPLY AND GRADUALLY ADD AND INCREASE. BE CONSTANTLY AWARE OF THE CLIENT'S CONDITION AS THE TREATMENT PROGRESSES. WHENEVER THE CLIENT FEELS LIGHT-HEADED OR DIZZY OR HAS A HEADACHE, IT'S TIME TO STOP.**

> **OVERALL CONTRAINDICATIONS:**
> - **Heart disease**
> - **Extreme high or low blood pressure**
> - **Any systemic disease, including immune disorders, cancer, diabetes, epilepsy, hemophilia**
> - **Pregnancy (particularly hydrotherapy and full body)**
> - **Areas of open wounds, lesions, infection, inflammation, edema (swelling), varicose veins, phlebitis, and other vascular problems**

SPA POINT

In general, when in doubt don't do it. Whenever there is a systemic disease or chronic problem obtain a physician's consent. Avoid doing too much of anything on a questionably healthy individual. The conservative approach is the safest and a good base from which to grow.

TREATMENTS FOR THE DAY SPA

The true day spa may include every kind of beauty-related service, from hair services to facial esthetics, nail care, and body care. The scope of this book will not include treatments for the face, hair, and nails except as they are related to specifically targeted spa-like treatments such as a seaweed scalp treatment, a special mud mask for the face, or a spa manicure or pedicure. Treatments will be described loosely. Each product line may have an interesting twist to a basic concept or a specialized treatment that may not be included here. Also, part of the fun of offering spa treatments is the ability to mix and match and come up with your own distinct combinations. Packages and combining will be discussed more fully in *Day Spa Operations*.

Remember that the three main concepts we'll be dealing with are exfoliation, full-body, and spot treatments. Rough times will be listed for treatments. These times will vary according to the goal of the treatment, combinations thereof, and the manner in which sales are being done. The most important thing to remember is to always allow time for selling products. It must be said again and again that the money in this business is in the retail. If you don't have enough time to allow for a retail presentation, you will not only lose money in retail sales, but also do your client a disservice. The home care follow-up is vital to spa success. See also chapter 13 and *Day Spa Operations*.

. . . .

SPA POINT

Exfoliation, body wraps, mud, seaweed, and essential oils are typical components of spa treatments. These may be mixed for the optimum treatments to make your spa unique. Manufacturers have their own game plan, treatment concepts, and ingredient innovations. It's imperative to research various product lines for more details on a specific treatment.

. . . .

Exfoliation

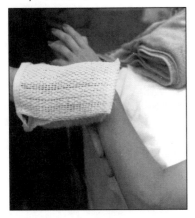

FIGURE 8-1 *Exfoliate dead surface skin in order to stimulate circulation.*

DRY BRUSH
This involves the use of a loofah, brush, washcloth, or sponge to exfoliate dead surface skin in a mechanical manner (Figure 8-1). Normally this is a prelude to a body treatment of some kind and, as such, is not a chargeable service (normally 10 minutes in a full-body treatment). If, however, the dry brush is a treatment by itself with just a finishing lotion and enough time is given to it (30 minutes), then it can become a chargeable service. The main purpose is to stimulate circulation (see chapter 9 for details).

SALT GLOW
Special salt is mixed with an oil or liquid soap to exfoliate the entire body or just an area for a spot treatment (Figure 8-2). This treatment when done alone on the full body followed by a lotion constitutes a chargeable service (30 minutes). When done as part of a spot treatment, such as a spa pedicure or manicure where salt is a quick exfoliant (5 minutes), it's normally included in

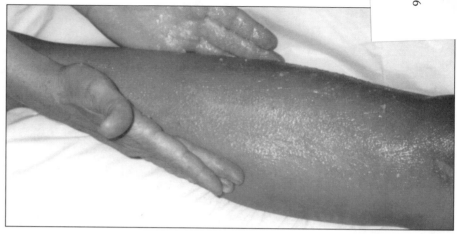

FIGURE 8-2 *Salt glow treatments can exfoliate dead surface skin on the entire body, or on a specific area of the body.*

the price of the treatment. The purpose is to exfoliate dead skin to allow for better penetration of moisturizers and conditioners (see chapter 9).

Salt glows are popular destination spa treatments and the term *salt glow* is easily understood by the consumer so is, therefore, easier to market. Some technicians will combine a dry brush tool such as a loofah with the salt mixture for extra exfoliation. Be careful not to overdo. The exfoliation procedure alone when done in conjunction with a manicure or pedicure will constitute a spa manicure or spa pedicure. Normally salt is not used on the face. Also if salt is being used, the client should not wax or shave for one to two days prior to treatment.

BODY POLISH

Salt or any abrasive substance or granular scrub can be used as a body polish (Figure 8-3). The term is used to separate an exfoliation with salt or other substance even though you could use salt to do this. Normally in

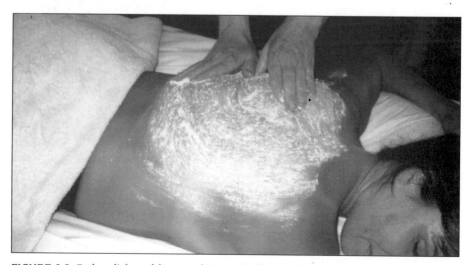

FIGURE 8-3 *Body polishes exfoliate, condition, and soften the skin at the same time.*

body polishes, the product has a cream base with granules of the abrasive to exfoliate and condition or soften the skin at the same time. Body polishes may take a little more time than salt glows depending on the texture and removal process. Body polishes may be done in 30–45 minutes as a treatment alone or in 5–10 minutes with spot treatments. Leah Kovitz, formerly of Canyon Ranch, developed a very special body polish called the Parisian Body Polish, which utilizes crushed pearls. This is an elegant, luxurious body polish. Many body polishes should not be used on the face. Be sure to check with your manufacturer. If the polish is aggressive, shaving or waxing for a day or two before should be avoided.

ENZYME AND AHA DISSOLVING EXFOLIANTS

Even though some proteolytic enzymes such as papaya can dissolve dead skin in a quite effective and aggressive way, we should not actually call these peels. They are, but when the consumer thinks of a peel the normal thought process is a chemical peel such as TCA (trichloracetic acid) or phenol. These are not recommended for use by a beauty practitioner. We do, however, often use the popular AHAs (alpha hydroxy acids) such as glycolic acid and lactic acid, and some BHAs (beta hydroxy acids) such as salicylic acid. The AHAs are effective in dissolving dead cells. The difference between scrubs and AHAs or enzymes is simply that scrubs and polishes abrade the dead cells off and the AHAs and enzymes dissolve dead cells that are ready to be sloughed off (Figure 8-4). Although the enzyme type is more aggressive, there can be more skin irritation due to the mechanical action of rubbing too much. Some manufacturers are now including AHAs in abrasive scrubs. This may be redundant so choose and use carefully. Waxing or shaving should be avoided for one or two days before.

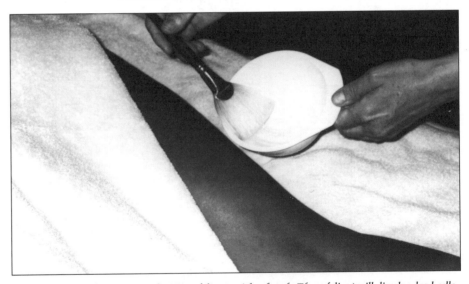

FIGURE 8-4 *Apply enzyme and AHA exfoliants with a brush. The exfoliant will dissolve dead cells that are ready to be sloughed off.*

. . . .

SPA POINT

Exfoliants allow whatever else is used in treatment to be more effective. Mechanical products such as scrubs, brushes, etc. abrade dead cells off, whereas AHAs and enzymes dissolve dead cells. They are all important to allow the skin to be more conducive to absorbing nutrients.

. . . .

Full-Body Treatments

FULL-BODY SEAWEED MASK

Seaweed powders are normally mixed with water to form a pancake-batter-like consistency. Different combinations of seaweed may be used for different effects on the body. Some companies have the seaweed in an already mixed wet form. The mixture is applied to the entire body over a conditioner, lotion, or ampoule if desired. The entire body may be covered or the stomach, breasts, and buttocks may be eliminated according to the desire of the client and technician. The body is then wrapped in foil or plastic as has been discussed in the previous chapter and the client rests for 20–30 minutes (Figure 8-5).

NOTE: *We do not recommend ace bandage or plastic wraps of legs as these can be too constrictive and hence dangerous. We use only blanketing wraps.*

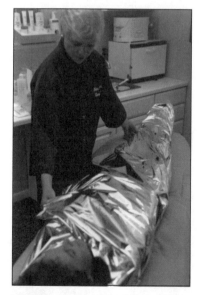

FIGURE 8-5 *Wrap the body in foil or plastic so that the client is warm and comfortable.*

Full-body seaweed masks often work with essential oils added to the mask for different effects on the body. A variety of results can be obtained based upon the essential oils included, from calming to stimulating to detoxifying. The full-body seaweed mask treatment normally takes about 60 minutes. Allow 15 minutes between clients for cleanup and sales.

FULL-BODY MUD MASK

There are a variety of muds available on the market, from sea-based muds to clay muds and fango (volcanic ash and sulfur from Italy), from moor mud (the noted Remy Laure Moor Mud from the boggy moors) to glacial mud. Depending on the mud, the effects may be to cleanse and draw out impurities, to condition and mineralize the body, or to just soften and hydrate the skin. Mud is normally warmed in a plastic container (some suggest avoiding metal bowls or microwave heating) in hot water or in a double boiler (if available) before application. The manufacturer will make specific recommendations. The mud is applied thickly (Figure 8-6) and the body is then wrapped in plastic or foil and allowed to rest for 20–30 minutes. It's wise not to apply mud on the palms of the hands in case the client has to scratch or grab something, or the feet in case the client has to go to the restroom. A full mud treatment normally takes about 60 minutes. Allow 15 minutes between clients for cleanup and selling.

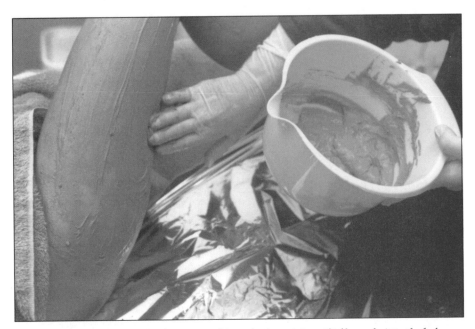

FIGURE 8-6 *Once the mud has been warmed in a plastic container, thickly apply it to the body.*

HERBAL BODY WRAP

Linen or muslin sheets are heated and soaked in a machine called a hydroculator (temperature inside hydroculator is about 150–175 degrees F). Herbal pouches or bags of herbs and essential oil essences are placed in the hydroculator for the effects desired. The body is first covered with towels or rubber sheets and then the linen or muslin sheets are laid over this (Figure 8-7). The body is then wrapped in sheets and blankets and allowed to rest for 20 minutes. A cool wet cloth is applied to the client's forehead during the treatment and changed often. This treatment can be done in 30

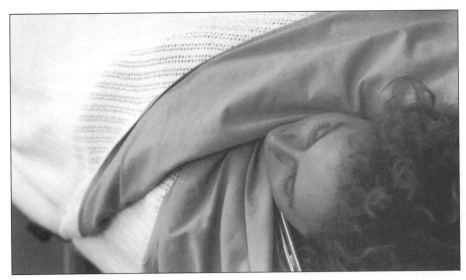

FIGURE 8-7 *For a herbal body wrap, the body is wrapped with towels and covered with muslin or linen sheets.*

minutes. Allow 5–10 minutes between clients for cleanup and selling. Understand that the wet sheets are heavy and very hot. Thick long rubber gloves must be worn by the technician. The average technician can do only four to six wraps a day without tiring from the weight of sheets. The linen sheets normally do not touch the client's body directly.

PARAFFIN BODY WRAP

Paraffin when applied to the body forms an occlusive mask with heat. This helps the body to perspire and the trapped moisture absorbs into the skin with whatever nutrients have been put on the skin first or from the oils in the paraffin. Paraffin may be used alone or mixed with mud, as in a parafango mud, or with seaweed as in a paraffin seaweed. Some technicians paint paraffin directly on the body with a large paint brush. It is more hygienic and effective to take large strips of gauze, dip them in the paraffin, and mold them to the different parts of the body being treated (Figure 8-8). Several layers will be applied, the more layers, the greater the heat and the longer it will last. After applying three to five layers of paraffin-soaked gauze, the body is wrapped in plastic or foil and allowed to rest for 15–20 minutes. When the paraffin has cooled off, there is no need to keep it on the body, so removal is appropriate. In a full-body treatment, allow 60 minutes for completion and 15 minutes between clients for cleanup and sales.

Paraffin is commonly done as a spot treatment for hands and feet, the back or the face. Basically the procedure will be the same, but in the case of hands and feet, there are insulated or electric mittens and booties available to facilitate the holding of heat. Do not turn on the electric booties or mittens.

BODY MASSAGE

Body massage is probably the most basic and most important day spa treatment available and the most appreciated by the client. There are many varia-

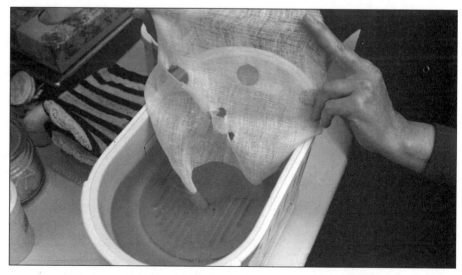

FIGURE 8-8 *The gauze has been customized to fit the client's body before dipping in the paraffin.*

tions from the basic Swedish to sports, deep tissue, Shiatsu, aromatherapy, manual lymph drainage (MLD), and reflexology. Sometimes the more sophisticated massages, such as aromatherapy and manual lymph drainage, have an extra charge. Massages are normally charged by the half-hour or hour but are, in actuality, 25 and 55 minutes respectively. Most spas book massages on the hour and half-hour. This will vary somewhat when done in combination with spa body treatments, which is, of course, the desired goal.

FULL-BODY FACIAL

This is a treatment similar to a facial treatment. The treatment includes cleansing, exfoliation, steam, extractions on the back if necessary, massage (half- or full hour), mask, and finishing lotion. This is a very popular treatment and can be booked for 60 or 90 minutes. Allow 15 minutes for cleanup and selling. The steam portion of this can be done with a facial steamer, hot towels, or a steam shower beforehand.

BODY TANNING/BRONZING

Of great popularity recently and a good way to convince your client to avoid sun as much as possible, this treatment consists of a full-body exfoliation and then application of a tanning emulsion. The tanning product is normally included in the treatment. The technician uses the retail bottle to apply and then gives the client the rest to take home to maintain the tanning process. The exfoliation is essential to make sure that the tanning solution goes on smoothly. The results of the tanning are much more effective when applied by the professional in the salon with the follow up done at home by the client. This treatment can be done in 30–45 minutes depending on the client, skin condition, and product being used. Allow 5–10 minutes for cleanup and selling.

. . . .

SPA POINT

There is a vast array of combinations of treatments for the whole body. Most include some kind of mask and wrap to seal in the nutrients, cause perspiration, and stimulate the circulation.

. . . .

Spot Treatments

Sometimes spot treatments are just mini versions of the full-body treatment. Sometimes specific spot treatments are done in conjunction with a full-body treatment. For example, a special firming bust treatment may be done underneath the full-body seaweed or mud mask. The advantage of doing some spot treatments with a full-body treatment is the fact that often the area is covered with a mud or seaweed mask and wrapped just as in a full-body. So if the client is having mud or seaweed applied and then is being wrapped up and allowed to rest for 20–30 minutes, why not combine a couple of extra spot treatments that are similar at the same time? Coordination of additives to masks, essential oils, or ampoule applications; types and lengths of massages; and the mask format will determine when you can or cannot mix.

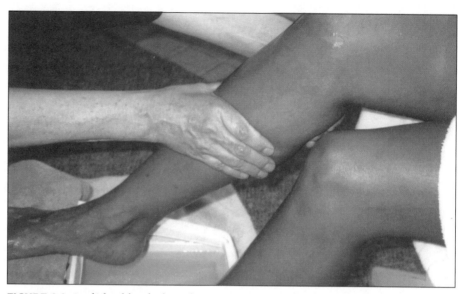

FIGURE 8-9 A *whirlpool foot bath can be an important part of a day spa pedicure.*

Remember to combine like treatments. If you're doing a mud mask and the firming bust treatment calls for a mud mask, then you can likely mix the two. If a product is supposed to be applied and quickly wiped off, then you wouldn't want to put it under a mask that is supposed to sit for 20 minutes. Refer to your manufacturer for specific guidelines on what mixes with what, and see chapter 12 for procedures.

SPA MANICURE, SPA PEDICURE

Many things can be done in a regular manicure or pedicure to qualify the treatment as "spa." This can be as simple as exfoliating with a scrub or enzyme. It may be because a whirlpool-type foot bath is used and essential bath oils are included in the water (Figure 8-9). It may be because the massage is performed with essential oils mixed in. And finally, the hands/arms and feet/legs may be enveloped in mud or seaweed masks and wrapped up just like for the full-body. The wrap for hands and feet should last no more than about 10 minutes. The important characteristic that makes the manicure or pedicure a spa treatment is the emphasis and specific steps developed for the treatment. It will normally add anywhere from 15 to 30 minutes for a regular manicure or pedicure, so pricing should follow suit. As mentioned previously, paraffin can also be included for an additional charge. Paraffin alone should not really constitute a spa treatment since it's been used in salons for years. But if exfoliation, aromatherapy massage, or special essential oil baths are done, then the paraffin falls quite well into the spa treatment category.

SPA HAND AND FOOT TREATMENT

This treatment would concentrate on exfoliation and massage, most likely with aromatherapy additives and perhaps a mud or seaweed mask. The important difference in this and the spa manicure or spa pedicure is the fact that the nails aren't treated. This treatment will be centered on the skin and underlying tissues, not on the glamour side. Estheticians, for example, will often do spa hand and foot treatments even though they don't know how to do a manicure or pedicure. If doing both hands and feet, allow 30 minutes total. If only doing hands or feet, this should be about a 10–15 minute add-on to another treatment. Otherwise it is not cost effective to block the time just for a 15-minute treatment. It would then be better to book a spa manicure or pedicure instead. Allow 5–10 minutes for cleanup and selling.

SCALP TREATMENT OR SCALP AND NECK TREATMENT

This is a great treatment for the cosmetologist or spa technician to perform. A great scalp treatment will naturally ruin the hairdo so it's important to be able to wash and restyle it. The hair should at least be shampooed and blown dry. The client must be informed in advance if styling can't be done. This isn't to say that styling can't be an extra charge. Spas price scalp treatments alone or in conjunction with a shampoo/style. Scalp treatments are designed to really clean, condition, and soften the scalp. The treatment is invigorating and refreshing. Most often a scalp treatment includes massage with oil or essential oils and a cleansing and conditioning mask. This mask could be mud, seaweed, or any other mask appropriate for the goal. The massage should last about 15 minutes, the mask about 10 minutes. After the mask has been applied, the head may be steamed with a facial steamer, hot towels, or steam dryer if available. Sometimes, the head is covered with foil or plastic and then wrapped in hot towels to keep the heat in longer. The treatment time should be no more than 30 minutes. Allow 5–10 minutes for cleanup and sales.

CELLULITE

This is undoubtedly one of the most popular treatments for women. Cellulite is a constant battle and one without cure. The spa treatments available for cellulite reduction and control help but are not a panacea. Never claim eradication of the cellulite. We can only facilitate the control. Remember, cellulite control requires a concerted effort on the part of the client who must drink lots of water, eat a high fiber diet, get lots of active exercise, obtain treatments, and use products effective to help in the elimination. All of these facets must be involved in the cellulite control program; one alone will not reduce cellulite. Also, as you do cellulite treatments, be careful not to refer to them as slimming or weight-loss treatments. This is not under the scope of our licensure. At the present time, the FDA does not recognize EMS (electric muscle stimulator) devices for our use. All we're doing in cellulite treatment is to help the body rid itself of cellulite through the active stimulation of the circulation and elimination processes. This is effectively done with aggressive massage, stimulating oils, and mud and seaweed wraps.

The cellulite treatment normally consists of exfoliation, application of a substance that stimulates the circulation and metabolic processes, massage, and then a mud or seaweed mask (Figure 8-10). The wrap is done as

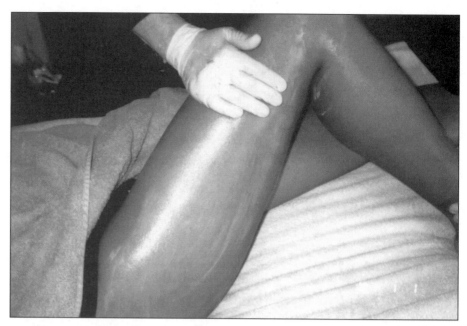

FIGURE 8-10 *Cellulite treatments are effectively done with aggressive massage, stimulating oils, mud wraps, and seaweed wraps.*

always and the client rests for about 20 minutes. The cellulitic areas are conditioned and moisturized after treatment. The entire treatment should normally be done in 30 minutes, 45 minutes at the most. Allow 10–15 minutes for cleanup, client instruction, and selling.

ANTISTRESS SPOT TREATMENT
This is a nebulous term for relieving stiff, sore, achy muscles. This is not a cure but just a relief. Some spas like to call it a muscle relaxation treatment.

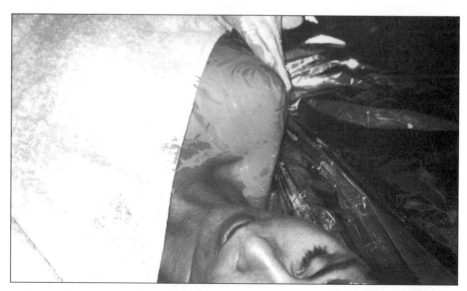

FIGURE 8-11 *Applying mud masks to the shoulder can be an effective antistress spot treatment.*

The area—shoulders, knees, lower back, neck, or wherever there is stress—is exfoliated and massaged well, and then treatment substances and the mud or seaweed masks are applied (Figure 8-11). Essential oils such as pine, rosemary, cinnamon, and thyme are very effective in stimulating the circulation to those areas and the massage relaxes the warmed muscles. The mask then furthers the warming, relaxing effects. The area is wrapped in foil or plastic as usual and allowed to rest for 15–20 minutes. The total treatment time should be about 30 minutes with 5–10 minutes for cleanup and sales. This is excellent to combine with a body massage or other full-body treatment.

FIRMING BUST TREATMENT

There are no treatments short of surgery that will increase or decrease the bust size. However, bust treatments are very effective for improving skin condition and texture, strengthening the pectoral muscles, and generally toning up the area. When the bust area is in better tone, there is a slight lifting effect that may be viewed by some as a sort of increase. It's not, but the lifting effect feels so. As shy as American women are about having bust treatments, if the truth be known, there probably isn't a soul out there who wouldn't like a better bustline. Additionally, a series of weekly bust treatments will dramatically improve any bust surgical procedure, and treatment is also good afterward when a physician calls for massage to keep an implant supple. The massage is part of the treatment and becomes a great marketable resource.

Though treatments are important, selling them is another story. If you find it difficult to sell bust treatments, begin by offering home care products. When the client gets used to the activity of applying them and seeing

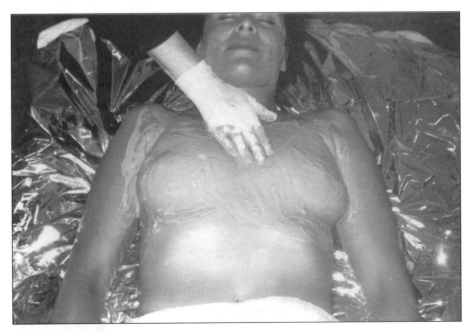

FIGURE 8-12 *Apply a stimulating product to the breasts, and massage.*

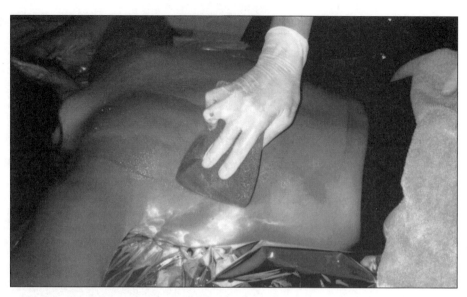

FIGURE 8-13 *Cleanse and exfoliate the back before extracting pustules and comedones.*

a minor result, it should then be fairly easy to get the client back into the spa for professional treatment. The treatment consists of a mild exfoliation followed by the application of a stimulating product (similar to that used in cellulite or stress relief treatments but milder) and massage (Figure 8-12). The massage is done on the soft tissue, avoiding the nipple area. A seaweed or mud mask is applied, and then the area is covered with foil or plastic. Some interesting thermal heating mineral clay masks and treatments are available. They warm, harden, and mold to the bust area and are highly effective. The treatment time should be under 30 minutes with 10–15 minutes allowed after for consultation, cleanup, and sales.

BACK TREATMENT OR BACK FACIAL
The back is a wonderful area for spot treatments. In fact, back facials have been done for many years as part of the esthetician's repertoire. As a spa concept, the main addition would be in the area of essential oils for aromatherapy massage and sea or mud masks. The client can't reach his/her own back well and this is an area of congestion, dead cell buildup, dryness, and itchiness, and is, therefore, a prime target for treatment. If your client base is one that attends many formal parties where women wear open-backed gowns, this will be a big seller.

Although the treatment may vary extensively, the basic concept follows: Cleanse, exfoliate, steam the back, and extract pustules and comedones if necessary (Figure 8-13). Perform a relaxing massage and apply a mud or seaweed mask. The back will be covered with foil or plastic and allowed to sit for 15–20 minutes. This treatment may be done in 30 minutes if the exfoliation or extraction processes are not long. Sometimes it is better to charge a little more and allow for a longer treatment. Book 1 hour for a 45-minute treatment. This will allow plenty of time for the best

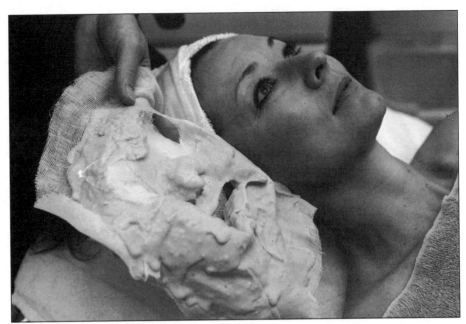

FIGURE 8-14 *Spa facials should include seaweed, mud, and/or aromatherapy, something that will relax the client while gently treating the face.*

treatment and great massage. A good back treatment will go far in selling your other spa services.

SPA FACIAL

This is an interesting term for a facial treatment that may concentrate on the mud or seaweed mask or include aromatherapy in the massage. In reality, facials have utilized all the spa-like substances for many years. But if the treatment highlights these concepts, there's nothing wrong with naming it spa facial. If you want to do a spa facial be sure to include seaweed, mud, aromatherapy—something that will make it more spa conducive (Figure 8-14). Remember, however, that most scrubs, salt, and other body exfoliants may be too strong for the face. Double check with the manufacturer.

. . . .

SPA POINT

Spot treatments are very much in demand. They are quick, easy, and profitable, particularly when done in conjunction with a full-body mask, massage, or other treatment. Of all the ones listed, probably the back, cellulite, and antistress are the most popular. Be sure some form of these are offered in your day spa.

. . . .

NOTE: *When combining treatments, it's usually best to do the hydrotherapy tub first, the body treatment, then the massage. Other showering devices would be used after the body treatment. The massage would be last.*

. . . .

TABLE OF TREATMENT TIMES

NOTE: *The following table is a rough guideline to assist you in planning your time and booking appointments. As a general rule, 30 extra minutes should be allowed with a first-time client and 15 minutes thereafter for cleanup and selling time. Also, remember that technically for every hydrotherapy treatment equal time should be allowed for resting. Therefore, to make the most of the time and still care properly for the client, try to book a treatment in combination with the hydrotherapy treatment. This will avoid unnecessary time loss.*

Treatment Name	Treatment Time	Wrap or Mask Waiting Time	Cleanup, Selling Time	Total Booking Time
Dry brush alone	30 minutes	none	5-10 minutes	45 minutes
Dry brush with treatment	10 minutes	none	5-10 minutes	depends on treatment
Salt/cond.	30 minutes	none	5-10 minutes	45 minutes
Salt with treatment	5 minutes	none	5-10 minutes	depends on treatment
Body polish	30 minutes	none	5-10 minutes	45 minutes
Body polish with treatment	5-10 minutes	none	5-10 minutes	depends on treatment
Enzyme or AHA	5-20 minutes	few minutes	5-10 minutes	30-45 minutes
Full-body seaweed	45 minutes	30 minutes	15 minutes	1 hour
Full-body mud	45 minutes	30 minutes	15 minutes	1 hour
Herbal wrap	30 minutes	20 minutes	5-10 minutes	30-45 minutes
Full-body paraffin	45 minutes	30 minutes	15 minutes	1 hour
Body massage	30 minutes or 1 hour	none	15 minutes	45 minutes or 1 hour
Body facial	1 or 1 1/2 hours	10-20 minutes	15 minutes	1 1/4 to 1 3/4 hours
Body tanning	30 minutes	none	5-10 minutes	45 minutes
Spa manicure/pedicure	15-30 minutes added to regular time	10-15 minutes if mask or wrap done	5-10 minutes	45 minutes
Hand/foot treatment	20-30 minutes	10-15 minutes if mask or wrap done	5-10 minutes	45 minutes
Scalp	30 minutes	10-15 minutes	5-10 minutes	45 minutes
Cellulite	30 minutes	15-20 minutes	15 minutes	45 minutes
Antistress	30 minutes	15-20 minutes	15 minutes	45 minutes
Bust	30 minutes	15-20 minutes	15 minutes	45 minutes
Back	30-45 minutes	15-20 minutes	15 minutes	45 minutes to 1 hour
Spa facial	normal facial time	10-15 minutes	15 minutes	1 hour to 1 1/2 hours

COMBINING TREATMENTS WITH HYDROTHERAPY

Any and all treatments can be combined with hydrotherapy and massage. It's best to consider a combination of two to three modalities at most until you know the client's tolerance level well. Combining or layering treatments effectively is what makes the whole spa concept so wonderful for the client and profitable for the salon. The following will represent a few of the common combinations. There are endless combinations and names. In *Day Spa Operations*, a great deal of emphasis will be put on packages and naming.

Please understand that these are merely a few suggestions on common combinations. You may devise your own.

Swiss Shower

Combine with:

1. Massage
2. Spot treatment and full-body treatment
3. Mud
4. Massage and paraffin

The regular or Swiss shower will be done after the treatment for warming, invigorating, and rinsing purposes. Ideally the shower should be close by. The treatment will be done in the treatment room not in the shower. They just book well together.

Vichy Shower

Combine with:

1. Salt glow
2. Mud
3. Seaweed

This is the best treatment combination for products that are hard to get off. It's great to do the treatment in the Vichy shower room and then make the Vichy shower part of the treatment as well as the rinsing device.

Steam Shower

Combine with:

1. Herbal wraps
2. Spot treatments
3. Aromatherapy massage

Again, the shower will be done after the treatment. Treatment will be done in a treatment room not in the shower.

Hydrotherapy Tub

Combine with:

1. Additives in the tub such as essential oils, seaweed, some muds, milk, bath salts, without underwater massage
2. Underwater massage followed by a mud or seaweed wrap
3. Massage, 30 minutes or 1 hour
4. Full-body mask and massage

Do not attempt to combine too many spot treatments and full-body treatments after a tub treatment, particularly if essential oils have been added or if underwater massage is performed. This client will likely overtire. Keep the combinations simple with hydrotherapy tub treatments. The tub itself should be the highlight. A simple massage is probably the best combination. If the client is very healthy, a massage and full-body mask is great.

. . . .

SPA POINT

The combination of hydrotherapy and treatment greatly intensifies the effect of either by itself. Do not overtreat the client. It's safer to do fewer combinations until you know how your client handles it all.

. . . .

SCHEDULING

The most important and most difficult part about developing a good spa program is the scheduling. A major mistake most spas make is to book appointments back to back. If you have assistants and cleanup people as well as counter retailers, this is fine. But if your technician is to do the cleanup, get ready for the next client, consult with the existing client, and sell products you must allow time for this to take place. The retail sales will suffer horribly if you don't allow enough time. For a first-time client, an extra half-hour should be allowed for good consultation and sales. Thereafter, at least 15 minutes is necessary between appointments, and more should be allowed if hydrotherapy and wet rooms are involved. Cleaning a wet room and tub can take a good 15 minutes alone. When your operation becomes quite busy, the addition of an assistant to clean up and prepare for the next client is a natural money maker for you. Remember that your big profits are not in service but in product sales.

Synopsis

The treatments listed in this chapter are just the basics. From here additives, naming, packages, and combinations make your spa unique and interesting. As eager as you may be to have a client sample everything, be careful not to combine too many services together, particularly if hydrotherapy is involved, especially with a tub and underwater massage.

Review

1. What is necessary to make body treatments successful?

2. What are some common contraindications of body treatment?

3. Why is a salt glow good to offer in a day spa?

4. Can spa treatments cure cellulite? What can be expected?

5. Name the full-body treatments discussed in this chapter.

6. What are the three most popular spot treatments?

7. How does hydrotherapy in combination with treatments affect the treatment?

CHAPTER 9
Exfoliation

OVERVIEW

The term *exfoliation* is commonly used to mean the removal of dead skin cells. According to Webster's *Ninth New Collegiate Dictionary*, exfoliate is defined as, "1: to split into or give off scales, laminae, or body cells 2: to come off in thin layers or scales..." So our terminology is quite accurate. It has only been in recent years that this term has been popularized to the consumer. Now when a consumer hears the word exfoliant, it is generally well understood to mean dead skin removal.

REASONS FOR EXFOLIATION

The important question to consider is, why remove dead skin? Isn't there supposed to be a layer of dead skin on the surface to protect us? Isn't it often called the dead skin layer or horny layer after the dried up keratin on the surface? The answer to these questions is yes. The problem we have is an overabundance of dead skin cells. This overabundance can cause the skin to clog, comedones and pustules to form in areas where they are prone to occurring, dryness and flakiness to occur. In recent years, researchers have discovered that often the culprit in oily acne skin is not really chocolate and similar substances, but rather a phenomenon called hyperkeratinization and clogging. This simply means that the skin has an overabundance of dead cells and it clogs up with natural body oils, dirt, and debris. The consumer is now becoming more aware of this and the need to remove the dead cells in order to keep the skin from clogging.

But all of what has been discussed so far connotes facial care. What about dead cells on the body? We are accustomed to thinking about cleansing the face and removing dead cells, but wouldn't you think the body needs it just as much? Well, it does for the most part. The only real advantage the body has is that it's covered most of the time and oil production isn't as prolific. However, removal of dead skin cells from the body is just as important. This removal can be done in a number of ways at home and at the day spa, and a number of different types of tools and agents facilitate the dead cell removal. But before going into the treatments, what does exfoliation provide? Exfoliation...

...perks up skin color and clarity.

...unclogs the follicles and pores.

...allows the skin to breathe better.

...allows moisturizers, lotions, serums etc. to penetrate the skin better.

…improves the skin's texture and makes it smoother.

…stimulates the skin's overall functions and increases circulation.

Exfoliation, therefore, is the first and most important treatment to be performed in a viable skin and body care treatment. The subsequent treatment goals will be greatly enhanced by the exfoliation process. The problem with exfoliation is that because it's so effective and obvious, it's quite easy to overexfoliate. People who have used abrasives on their face daily for years have shown to have a skin thickening with time. This winds up being unattractive and, in fact, can make the skin look quite leathery in a way similar to inveterate sun bathers over decades of sun abuse. It is important to remember at all times that exfoliation is good but not too much too often. It's better to be on the conservative side of treatment. Additionally, depending on the exfoliant and how it is used, it's possible to increase the skin's own sensitivity to other topical substances, so caution is advisable with all exfoliants. This is why exfoliation should be under the control and direction of a licensed professional.

. . . .

SPA POINT

Exfoliants are the first step in viable treatments in order to remove dead skin so that the subsequent treatments will be more effective, to smooth and improve skin texture. However, overexfoliation is not good and with time can increase skin sensitivity and cause skin thickening. Therefore, exfoliation should be under the control and direction of a licensed professional.

. . . .

TYPES OF EXFOLIANTS

In spa treatments we will be dealing with two basic types of exfoliants, mechanical exfoliants and enzymatic or dissolving exfoliants. We generally do not use chemical peels such as trichloracetic acid or resorcinol. These are chemical peels normally under the control of a physician. In reality, they aren't needed for normal body treatment. Let's look at what's available in mechanical and dissolving exfoliants.

Mechanical Exfoliants

Mechanical exfoliants are called this because they normally involve a mechanical process of rubbing to accomplish the exfoliation. These work from an abrasive standpoint, the substance and the hands in a rubbing format.

DRY BRUSH

Brushes, much like a hairbrush, stimulate the circulation and buff off dead cells. Nylon mitts, loofah sponges and mitts, and abrasive cloths are all designed to work like the brush to remove dead cells (Figure 9-1). Most brushes are made of natural goat's hair or other bristle. Some are more

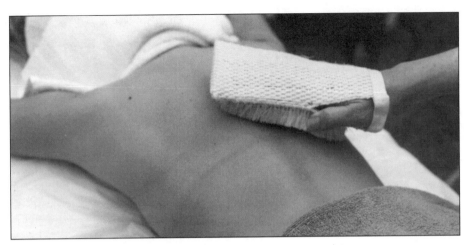

FIGURE 9-1 *Exfoliating the back with an abrasive mitt.*

abrasive than others, and in different situations you may choose to use one tool over another. For those with facial equipment, the brush device on your machine may also be used with the larger body brush attachment if desired. They are usually used as a lead-in to a body treatment to stimulate the blood flow and to make the treatment work better. Or it can be done by itself as a type of exfoliating massage.

Whether doing it as a lead-in to a treatment or by itself as a stimulating massage, it should be done ideally on dry skin. If the skin is too sensitive, it may be done on wet skin. In either case, the massage movements should be gentle and rhythmical, but not irritating or uncomfortable. A slight erythema (reddening) of the skin is fine, but don't overdo it. Dry brushing when done alone as a massage treatment can be done slowly and in more detail, taking as long as 30 minutes for the whole body. When dry brushing prior to treatment, the whole procedure should take only about 10 minutes. Dry brushing before certain spot treatments is effective as well, particularly before a cellulite treatment. The dry brushing should take place immediately before the application of the cellulite treatment products and mask.

PROCEDURE

1. With the client lying on the back, the dry brushing begins with the foot (top and bottom) and proceeds up the front and sides of the leg. You can also brush the back first before client lies down.

2. The client is slightly turned now to dry brush the back of the leg, buttocks, and up one half of the back.

3. The upper shoulders and arms are brushed.

4. The back of the neck, chest (very gently), and stomach (if desired) are brushed. The bust area is not dry brushed. When brushing the stomach, remember to go in a clockwise direction.

5. Move to the foot of the other leg and repeat the entire process.

NOTE: *Ideally all brushing movements should follow your typical effleurage movements in a directional movement toward the heart.*

Another nice alternative is to dry brush the back while the client is sitting up before lying down.

SANITATION

Even though the client normally wasn't wet down for this treatment, the brushes, loofah, mitts, or whatever cloth was used must be thoroughly cleaned, disinfected, and dried between clients. This means that you should have several sets ready for a day's work. It takes a while for the brushes to dry.

SALT

As previously stated, you are not to work with plain table salt. It's very abrasive and can easily burn a client. Normally, special salts are used, often sea salt or Dead Sea salt. Be sure the salt is smoothly refined and comfortable for use on the client. There may be some differences between manufacturers, but most salt should not be used alone dry. Also, keep in mind that when doing most exfoliating treatments but particularly with salt, you don't want the client to wax or shave for two days prior to the treatment. Salt should be mixed with a liquid substance to make it move and glide over the skin easily (Figure 9-2). If showering facilities are available it's nice to mix salt with a bath gel liquid soap or, if not, with a disappearing massage oil. After the massage oil disappears, the salt residue can be dusted off the body.

A salt glow or salt exfoliation can be done as a treatment by itself. When doing a salt glow as a single treatment, the treatment will always end with the application of a body lotion and quick penetrating massage. If the salt is done with another treatment, it's still charged for but the procedure is done more quickly and is not quite so detailed. The amount of salt to solvent depends on the delicacy of the skin and whether the client is hairy. Use less salt for delicate skin. Use extra oil or liquid soap for men with a lot of hair. Some technicians like to use a loofah mitt with the salt mixture but in most cases this is too harsh and uncomfortable for the client.

PROCEDURE

1. Put 2–4 tablespoons of salt in a bowl with 1/4 cup oil or shower gel. For stronger exfoliation, add more salt. For delicate skin reduce salt. For men, double the oil or shower gel amount to increase slip on hairy areas. Salt plus oil should be used where shower is not readily available or not desired. Application in oil and dusting off salt residue takes more time than showering. Salt plus shower gel soap should be used only when showering off. Otherwise the soap will dry out the skin. Shower gel or soap may be a matter of personal choice or variation for regular clients when showering is always the rinsing method.

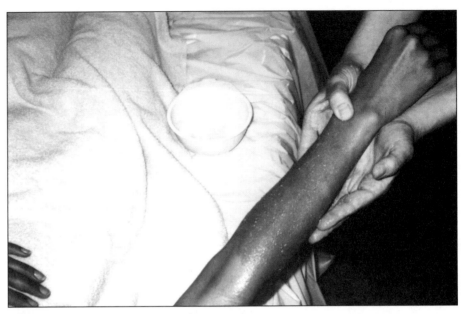

FIGURE 9-2 *Salt glow treatments slide over the skin and exfoliate the dead surface cells.*

2. Normally plastic covers a bed covered with a blanket, sheet, bath towel. If dusting the salt off, the plastic will be rolled off under the client. If showering, the plastic will be removed while the client is showering.

3. The application procedure will be the same as listed above for dry brushing starting with the feet and moving up. Again, if desired, the back may be done before the client lies down.

4. The client is either led to the shower to rinse off or is dusted off with dry towel. In both cases the plastic is removed. Client should be lying on a clean dry towel over a sheet.

5. After rinsing or dusting, the client will be rubbed down and massaged with a finishing lotion, oil, or cream. The treatment is finished. If salt is being done before a body wrap, for example, the beginning of the body treatment will begin when the client returns from the shower or when the plastic has been removed. The body treatment will end also with a body lotion so it is not necessary to apply lotion at this point.

BODY POLISH

The term *body polishing* can be used for any form of granular scrub. It's advisable to use this term for scrubs to differentiate from salt rubs, even though technically salt could be considered a body polish as well. Body polishes are scrubs containing some type of grain—polyethylene balls, pumice, oatmeal, ground-up nuts, and others. (Figure 9-3). There are myriad different types of body polishes. As mentioned previously, the Parisian Body Polish of Leah Kovitz is made up of crushed pearls. The exfoliating granules can make a big difference in the comfort level of the client. The cream base that it's in will also make a difference. If the granules are harsh, the base should be heavy and creamy. If the granules are more delicate, the base could even be a liquid shower gel. Look at various scrubs on the market to find the ones that suit your purposes.

If you plan to use a scrub on the face, be sure it's a very gentle one, particularly if it's available for retail. I personally do not like any granular scrubs for the face because I feel most clients tend to be too aggressive with them. Some scrubs are difficult to use on men and some are much too abrasive for delicate skin. Choose carefully and use gently. The degree of pressure and amount of rubbing will largely influence the strength of the treatment. As with salt, the body polish can be added to another treatment or be a treatment alone. Similar to salt, the treatment will end with a body lotion or conditioner.

PROCEDURE

1. Be sure the bed is set up with a blanket, sheet, and plastic sheet. The client will lie on the plastic sheet.

2. Take approximately 4–6 tablespoons of the scrub out of the jar, replace the cap, and work out of a bowl. The amount varies dramatically from supplier to supplier. Again use more for men, less for delicate skin.

3. The application procedure will be the same as for dry brushing. This time, however, if the scrub is quite gentle, you may choose to do the bust area carefully (always avoid the nipples). Adjust pressure and amount according to the body and product being used.

4. After the entire body is polished, the client will shower off the scrub and residue. Soap is not normally recommended to use in the showering.

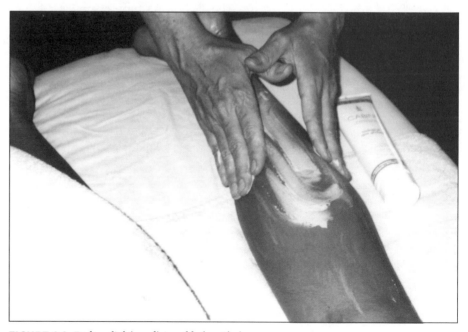

FIGURE 9-3 *Body polish (scrub) is rubbed on the leg.*

5. The plastic is removed and the client is placed on a fresh, clean towel for the final application of body lotion. If a body or spot treatment is to follow, do not apply lotion at this point but begin the other treatment.

NOTE: *Body polishes do well in wet rooms where the Vichy shower can easily rinse the residue off. It is rather difficult although not impossible to remove body polishes in a dry environment. You will normally want to use hot towels to remove the polish and residue.*

. . . .

SPA POINT

Mechanical exfoliants are very popular and give a great "spa" aura. The dry brush technique is used most often when a client is having another body treatment and is not purchasing a salt glow or body polish to rev up the skin. Ideally, salt will be the most popular in the spa because it's not retailed, which brings the client back. Most body polishes are also retailed so they are good for home care follow-up. It's great to have both for variation for the frequent spa client.

. . . .

Enzyme or Dissolving Exfoliants

Dissolving exfoliants comprise two concepts, one being the proteolytic enzymes such as lipo amino acids or papaya enzymes. The other one is part of the families of AHAs (alpha hydroxy acids) or fruit acids, and BHAs (beta hydroxy acids) such as salicylic acid. The potential advantage of dissolving exfoliants over the mechanical ones lies in the lack of rubbing necessity. For example, if someone has recently had a face-lift you wouldn't want to rub the face with a scrub but could easily paint on an enzyme or AHA and then delicately rinse it off without much skin movement at all. Depending on the product, the dissolving type are normally stronger than mechanical exfoliants. They work more aggressively at dissolving dead cells but don't overstimulate the skin from an abrasion standpoint. The mechanical exfoliants work aggressively from a rubbing standpoint, hence can irritate the skin more than dissolving exfoliants. This, of course, depends entirely on the different strengths of the various products compared. This is a bit of an oversimplification. Look to your manufacturers for specifics of their products. Many manufacturers carry both and recommend both for different purposes. Let's have a look at the dissolving exfoliants now.

ENZYMES

Enzymes have been popular for years in two formats—wash-off type and rub-off type. These have often been called rub-off peels. They are not peels, but the term was used to describe the effect of dead cell removal through the dissolution of keratin by proteins. Then the residue to the substance along with the dead skin was rubbed off by the technician (Figure 9-4). This type of exfoliant is still quite popular and used often for the face as well as the body. Even with the rub-off type, some of these enzyme exfoliants can also be washed off if rubbing is too sensitizing for the skin. Most often even if you can't rub it off the face, rubbing the body will be quite tolerable. In many cases, if the enzyme is designed to wash off, you'll still achieve a great exfoliation without the redness or irritation from rubbing it off. Some manufacturers recommend using steam with the product, and many specifically state that the skin must be dry so that the protein can function at its best. Follow your manufacturer's direction on this.

Many of the enzyme exfoliants are a mixture of a number of herbs, which are often kept secret by the manufacturer to preserve the uniqueness of the treatment. The FDA does not require specific ingredient listing for a professional treatment, only for the retail products, so this secret can be kept if they desire. However, in case of an allergic reaction, this can be quite a problem. You may want to choose a product that lists the ingredients voluntarily anyway. The herbal combinations are often quite stronger than the more elementary rub-off type. The following directions will work for most rub-off types.

PROCEDURE

1. The bed will be set up as always with blanket, sheet, towel, then plastic.

2. Ideally the client will take a quick shower and wash with your shower soap/gel and dry off. The client will then lie on the table face up.

3. Using the same pattern as already described for dry brushing, apply the product. The amount of product that you will use depends on the manufacturer. It may be a cream in a tube or a powder that is mixed with water or a solvent. If it's a cream in a tube, you will use about 3–4 tablespoons on a normal size body. If it's a powder that needs to be mixed with water, make about 1/3 cup for the body.

4. Make a thin layer on a large section of skin. Segment in groups, for example, do the foot, then do the calf. If the product requires drying or setting up time, you can apply it to another area, come back and rub the first area off and apply more to the next area, come back and rub

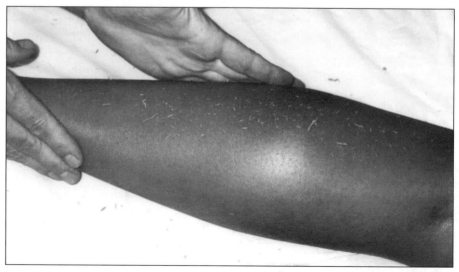

FIGURE 9-4 *The technician rubs the exfoliant and the dead surface cells off the body.*

off the second area, and so forth, alternating application and rub off. Do not attempt to do the entire leg in one movement. This can cause uneven drying, uneven exfoliation, and sometimes even irritation. Normally the product can be applied rather thinly and be effective, but be sure to check with your manufacturer. Areas that have a large dead cell buildup may require a thicker layer. Experiment until you know your best level of effectiveness.

5. Whether you should use a steamer to activate the product is up to the manufacturer. Sometimes using a facial steamer is difficult. If it is impractical and you have a steam shower or cabinet, apply product, let it set a few minutes, then have client sit in the steam area for the necessary time, and finally wash off the product and residue in the shower. You may still have to rub a little to be sure it's all off. But usually the client can remove it all in the shower with the help of a large body sponge, shammy, or other cloth.

6. Whether the product is rubbed or washed off, be sure the body is clean and plastic removed from the table. The client should again be lying on a clean dry towel. At this point, if the treatment is completed, a body lotion or cream should be massaged in to finish, or if another treatment is to take place next, proceed. As an example, if you're doing a full-body seaweed wrap with foil, the foil should have been placed on the table under the plastic or put on the table when the plastic is removed while the client is in the shower. In other words, if you know in advance that you will be doing the exfoliation and a seaweed wrap with foil, the bed should be set up in advance as follows: blanket, sheet, foil, plastic. If you don't want the client to lie directly on the plastic for the exfoliation, you may put a towel over the plastic but both must be removed as the exfoliant is removed.

AHAS AND BHAS
The advent of glycolic acid brought about a revolution in skin care treatment and exfoliation from a nonmedical standpoint. Whereas licensed beauty practitioners couldn't prescribe Retin A, we could use glycolic acid. As with all new things, time brings modifications and advancements. Now glycolic is most often teamed with other fruit acids. Some even use other acids entirely without glycolic. Some of the BHAs such as salicylic acid have a similar function without being as irritating. The variations often have to do with the intended goal for the product and treatment.

If you want to use AHAs and BHAs in treatment, that's fine. You'll need to obtain specific instructions from your manufacturer. The important thing to remember about the strength and intensity of the product is to look at the percentage, the pH, and whether it is self-timed or you have to time it with a watch. The higher percentages at very low pH (below 3) are much more aggressive. You will need to determine your level of safety and effectiveness with your manufacturer. Obviously the face cannot handle the stronger versions as well as the body, but the body is more sensitive than you may think. It's also wise to be sure the acid has humectants that moisturize the skin at the same time. Some manufacturers put low levels of AHAs in conventional exfoliants as well so there are many choices available.

PROCEDURE

1. The bed is set up the same as for enzyme exfoliants. The client is requested to shower and cleanse first and then lie on the bed face up.

2. The AHA/BHA is applied to the skin. The actual procedure here may vary dramatically between products. Some are painted on, some rubbed on, some applied in a paste (Figure 9-5). Follow the manufacturer's instructions for application, waiting time, and removal.

3. After the product has been removed by the recommended method, the client is returned to the bed for moisturizing or to continue with the next treatment in the same manner as step 6 in the enzyme treatment.

· ·

SPA POINT

Whether you are using a proteolytic (protein) enzyme or an AHA, the value of having a dissolving treatment that is strictly professional and not retailed has added benefits to the client as well as the salon. It keeps the client excited about results and also keeps that client coming in. Most enzyme type exfoliants should not be retailed.

· ·

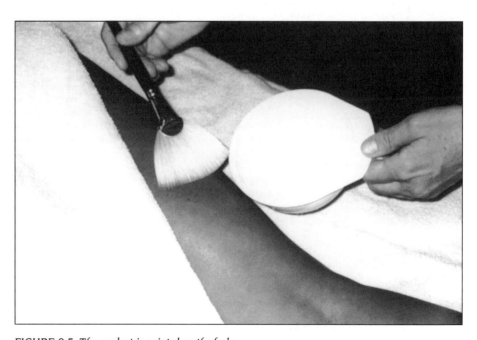

FIGURE 9-5 *The product is painted on the body.*

Contraindications

Overall, most exfoliants are quite safe to use on the skin. The client must, however, be taught how and when to use them at home. In the spa, the technician should be careful in the following situations:

- Do not use salt on open wounds or immediately after waxing or shaving. Body polishes and dissolving exfoliants also shouldn't be used immediately after waxing or shaving.

- Do not use exfoliants immediately after surgical procedures where the skin shouldn't be irritated or moved. Obtain physician's consent on when to treat.

- Do not rub sensitive areas; areas of telangiectasia (varicose veins, couperose); or areas of open wounds, infection, or inflammation.

- Exfoliants that are aggressive or require a rub-off procedure shouldn't be used on sensitive skin areas.

- Do not overexfoliate or rub too hard and fast.

- Do no exfoliation on sunburns.

. . . .

SPA POINT

Although exfoliants may be the star of the body show, do not overuse them or exfoliate too much. Normal caution should be used at all times.

. . . .

Synopsis

There is almost no treatment around that shouldn't be preceded by some type of exfoliation. The whole goal in exfoliation is to make the skin more product friendly for all the many treatments available. The exfoliation process is the first treatment the client receives in body work and often for the face as well. This gets the client off to a great start, and if you allow the client to feel the difference in her/his skin before and after the exfoliant, you will normally have yourself a hooked client. The exfoliation is often the most visually dramatic part of the treatment, at least from the client's viewpoint. You will see more as the treatment progresses, but this is the stage where the client is so readily impressed. If the client isn't asleep, be sure the benefits are pointed out right away. It will be most impressive.

Review

1. What does the word *exfoliant* mean?
2. Why are exfoliants valuable for the face and body?
3. Can you overexfoliate? If so, what happens?
4. What are the two types of exfoliants?
5. How do you choose between the two types?

CHAPTER 10
Mud Treatments

OVERVIEW

Perhaps nothing is more synonymous with spa concepts than the idea of using mud. In advertising of spas and spa services, what is most often pictured? When a body product company wants to feature a treatment, what scene is most often depicted? Yes, that's right, a full beautiful body slathered with smooth, silky, green mud.

From time immemorial, we have viewed mud with interest and curiosity. Mud has somehow always held images of soothing, drawing, and healing. In Rudyard Kipling's *Just So Stories*, do you remember how the elephant got his trunk? It was pulled and pulled by the crocodile, and after the great stretching, the elephant's child stuck his outstretched nose in the muddy waters of the great grey-green, greasy Limpopo River and "schlooped up a schloop of mud and slapped it on his head where it made a cool schloopy-sloshy mud cap all trickly behind his ears." What a great visual impression we have from that fairy tale, which dates back to the mid-1800s. The reality is that animals have forever bathed themselves in mud. Ancient civilizations such as the Romans have been depicted in frescoes using mud.

Mud holds much for us in the way of nutrition, healing, and skin care. What is it about mud that's so unique? And why do we use it?

· ·

SPA POINT

Mud epitomizes what a spa is all about to the consumer because it's been an integral part of spa concepts from ancient times. We even read books and see artistic representations of mud in applications, baths, and products so it is probably the most spa-like treatment available.

· ·

MUD IS REALLY CLAY

To research mud, you wind up studying clay. Clay is the substance; mud is simply wet and soupy clay. Another important word to understand in connection with clay and mud is *colloidal*, which is defined as "a substance that is in a state of division preventing passage through a semipermeable membrane, consists of particles too small for resolution through an ordinary light microscope, and in suspension or solution fails to settle out and diffracts a beam of light." In simpler terms this means that clays readily suspend in an emulsion with water or other liquid substance. This is one reason why fine-grained clays are so well used in cosmetics and other industries. Clays are considered colloidal substances.

Clays come from different soils and also from marine sediments. As a general rule marine-based clays have a higher mineral content than soil-based ones.

There are approximately eight types of clays: allophane; kaolinite; halloysite; smectite; illite; chlorite; vermiculite; and sepiolite, attapulgite, and polygorskite. Then there are mixtures of these.

· ·

SPA POINT

Marine-based clays generally have a higher mineral content than soil-based clays.

· ·

General Properties of Clays

Clays in general have certain properties. The category of clay may vary according to the specific mineral content and microscopic shape and structure of the clay particles. In general clays all have a strong affinity for positive or negative ion exchanges. This ionic activity has a great influence upon the type of clay and the economic uses for the clay. Clays readily react to temperature, especially heat. They can hold heat well, which makes them important in mask treatments and cosmetics. Because of the ionic organic compound's ability to hold or replace different compositions, clay also has a natural affinity for oil absorption. Thus it's used in processing oils and also in cosmetics designed to absorb oils.

Some clay minerals serve as catalysts for other organic materials and the reactions can cause change in colors. Organic clay minerals are used in paint, ink, and plastics.

Clay and water mix well and form a nongranular suspension unless sand is in the mixture (Figure 10-1). Thus the fine grains of clay form superior emulsions for masks. Also because of this smooth texture, in many cultures

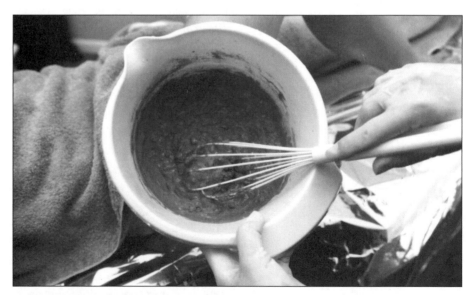

FIGURE 10-1 *Mix the clay and water in a plastic container.*

clay is mixed with water and drunk for health purposes. The Hunza population of the Himalayas claims that, to some degree, their long life and good health is due to drinking clay on a regular basis. Other holistic approaches to good health include drinking a solution of 1/2 teaspoon green clay to 8 ounces of water on a daily basis. It has been suggested that clay enriches the blood and stimulates circulation. Thus, clay is not to be used on anyone with high blood pressure.

Many clays are potential ores for aluminum and can be extracted. Most often, however, bauxite is used to extract aluminum. In general, clays are composed mainly of silica, alumina, water, iron, alkalis, and trace minerals. Minerals included may consist of calcium, magnesium, sodium, and potassium. Some may include small amounts of quartz, mica, feldspar, and iron oxides.

· ·

SPA POINT

Many believe that there is a kindred link between humans and mud. Mud is active, with great ionic exchange capability. Because of this, it is used in a number of industries. Mud has a very high mineral content that can be translated into therapeutic effects on the human body. The variety of clays and their different properties allow industry to use them as a natural renewable source of material for any number of products and functions.

· ·

CLAYS MOST OFTEN USED IN COSMETICS

Kaolinite (Kaolin)

From soils, this is a well-formed clay with six-sided flakes, normally a pure white (often called China clay), fine-grained clay. Kaolinite is used in masks and other cosmetics for deep cleansing, drawing, tightening, and toning. It has an overall mineralizing ability. In other industries, kaolinite is used in gasoline, porcelain, whiteware, ink, and organic plastics.

Illite/Chlorite

The composition of the two is similar, coming from soils and predominantly marine sediments. Illite is formed when potassium is added to kaolinite, and chlorite is formed when magnesium is added. This is common in marine-based soils. Soils containing illite and chlorite are better for agriculture due to their higher ion exchange properties and capacity to hold plant nutrients in the soil. These clays may also be used in cosmetics. Illite is used for brick, tile, stoneware, and glazed products.

Smectites

The composition forms broad undulating mosaic sheets and is found in some prairie, ash, and organic soils, but predominantly in volcanic ash. Bentonite is composed mostly of smectite clay and is very important as a cosmetic substance. The name comes from the area where it was found near Fort Benton, Montana. There are two types of bentonites. Sodium bentonite absorbs water and swells. This type is used to seal dams, with drilling muds, in ceramics, emulsions, soaps, pharmaceuticals, and paints. Calcium bentonites, popularly called "Fuller's earth," is a nonswelling clay that breaks down into a very fine granular aggregate and is used as an absorbent clay (great in masks for oily skin).

Another type of smectite mixture is magnesium aluminum silicate, known in cosmetic literature as "MAS." This mixture is the most versatile in cosmetics and will be listed on an ingredient label as MAS. MAS enhances water, oil, and grease absorption, helps keep emulsions from settling, and serves as a thickening agent. Since it is not easily affected by high temperatures or microbial damage, it improves the shelf life of a product.

It should be mentioned here that almost all clays are found in areas of hot springs and geysers due to the high mineral content of the soil. Hot spring clays are often referred to as fango muds, a term that originated in Europe. The spa at Montecatini, Italy, is perhaps most famous for fango muds. Fango mud is volcanic ash and sulfur, thus quite soothing and healing.

There are other highly mineralized muds that have gained notoriety over the years, such as moor mud from Austria, and glacial clay from a remote lagoon at the Pacific coast in Canada. Even though all clays have a high mineral content, specific clays may be more enriched and, therefore, have a greater value for different functions in cosmetics.

MAJOR CLAY MINERALS AND THE BODY

CALCIUM
Calcium strengthens bones and teeth and appears to be useful to increase the absorption and utilization of calcium in the body. It may also help control capillary permeability.

MAGNESIUM
Magnesium helps regulate and lower blood pressure. It is important in the metabolism and utilization of calcium and may help headaches. This is an essential mineral to maintain health.

POTASSIUM
Potassium helps balance electrolytes and works to prevent muscle cramps. It also releases energy from proteins, carbohydrates, and fats.

Calcium, magnesium, and potassium also act to regulate moisture.

TRACE MINERALS
Selenium is an antioxidant and interacts with vitamin E, iodine balances the thyroid, chloride assists in body fluid balance, iron enables red blood cells to carry and use oxygen, and zinc is required for all normal cell growth.

Minerals may further assist in maintaining and strengthening the body's immune system. Minerals and trace minerals also serve as catalysts for the utilization of vitamins in the human body and help keep skin moisture content balanced. (See also chapter 11 on Seaweed for more information.)

Clay Colors

In the cosmetic field, we tend to refer to clay by color as opposed to by name. The colors we most often deal with are green, red, yellow, and white. White is the kaolinite, used most for talc, deodorants, and masks. Green, which also is quite popular and appears to be the most active, is a smectite/chlorite or illite combination and is most often found in marine sediments. It is used for drinking, masks, and poultices. Red or rose clays are also smectite combinations and used mostly for deep cleansing, masks, packs, and smoothing rough skin. Yellow clay characteristics are similar to rose clay.

Another clay-based product, parafango, incorporates clay with paraffin to form a warm occlusive mixture that is most often used for heat transference. It causes greater dilation of blood vessels and increases circulation to the area. This is often used therapeutically for sore muscles and the like as a replacement for hot packs.

• •

SPA POINT

Calcium, magnesium, and potassium are very valuable minerals for overall health and body metabolism. They affect bones, blood pressure, and permeability, and also act as moisture regulators. This makes them very important minerals for skin and body treatments.

• •

TREATMENTS IN ESTHETICS

Mud has been used for centuries for therapeutic and beautification purposes for skin softening, for metabolic stimulation, and for simple relaxation. In some cases marine muds are used with similar results as seaweed. The mineralization may be similar but the feel, texture, and aura are different. In spas the world over, mud treatments will be sold over the seaweed treatments purely due to the aura around mud.

It's advisable to offer both seaweed and mud treatments. The combination and harmony of both enhances the activity of either and adds longevity to the facility's treatment capability. If you want to be classified as a true day spa, mud body treatments are a must.

General Information When Working With Clays

• Do not mix or store clay in metal containers. It will draw out the minerals.

• Do not overmix clay. Overmixing most clays affects their smooth structure and permeability.

• It is best to heat clay indirectly in a double boiler or in a container inside a heating unit with water. Microwave should not be used. Heat once and use. Do not reheat.

• Check with supplier regarding drain disposal requirements. Some muds may be used in a footbath, some may not.

• A Vichy shower is ideal for rinsing/treating simultaneously.

- Refer to manufacturer for more specific directions.

SUPPLIES NEEDED

Massage table or wet room table

1-2 cotton sheets (some clays stain, so green or grey sheets may be preferable)

3 bath sheets or large bath towels (also green/grey)

2 hand towels

1 bathrobe

1 electric bed warmer if allowable

1 regular cotton blanket

1 plastic sheet

2-4 body shammies, or 2 large body sponges, or 2-4 hand towels (should keep in hot towel cabinet for ready warm moist usage)

1 pair dry body brushes or mittens

1 large masking brush or spatula

1 large plastic or rubber mixing bowl

1 large wooden spoon for mixing

1 pitcher of cold water for client to drink as desired

EQUIPMENT NEEDED

Hot towel cabinet

Hydrotherapy tub, showers

Disinfectant

Cleansing products (including exfoliants)

Toning lotion/astringent

Essential oils/massage product

Muds (clays)

Body lotions/creams

Finishing powder

NOTE: *Be sure to check with your manufacturer regarding staining of linens and choose colors accordingly. Other specific supplies may be suggested by suppliers.*

Table Setup Over table drape electric bed warmer, regular blanket, bath sheet, cotton sheet, plastic sheet. Offer hand towel to client to cover breasts and have another hand towel as a diaper if necessary. If salt or scrub exfoliation precedes mud treatment, put another plastic sheet over the first plastic sheet to avoid necessity of showering after exfoliation is completed.

Client Preparation Preparation varies according to the selected treatment. If a full-body treatment is to be done, it is always best to have the client shower beforehand. It is also easier to perform the treatment if the client is nude and coverage is provided by sheets and towels over areas not exposed for treatment. The need for diaper and breast towel is determined by the client and technician. If the treatment being done is a local or spot treatment, that area must be exposed and precleansed.

MUD TREATMENTS

NOTE: *The treatment procedures for spot treatments will normally follow a pattern similar to the full-body mask or wrap. Variances may occur in choice of treatment products and essential oils, amount of time left on skin, and removal techniques. Therefore, the full-body treatment will be listed first.*

Full-Body Mud Treatment

GOAL OF TREATMENT
The goal of a full-body mud treatment may vary somewhat according to the client and other products used. As a general rule, mud treatments encourage increased blood circulation, absorb impurities from the skin, soften skin, and improve surface moisturization. A moisturizing mud would be used in this type of treatment. If exfoliation has been done, the effects of the mud are further heightened. To condition the body, a series of weekly treatments for 3–6 weeks is beneficial.

INDICATIONS FOR TREATMENT
All normal healthy individuals may receive treatments. Client must complete health history chart prior to treatment.

NOTE: *Full-body mud treatments can be difficult and time consuming if a shower or Vichy shower is not available. The ideal location for mud treatment is the Vichy shower room. If using a wet room, obviously electric bed warmers and blankets are not used. If the table isn't padded appropriately for a wet room, a foam mattress used in swimming may be used but covered with sheets. If using Vichy shower, technician will most likely get wet doing this treatment. Dress accordingly.*

PROCEDURE
1. Client should be placed on properly draped table after showering. Client should lie on back. Be sure client is immediately carefully covered.

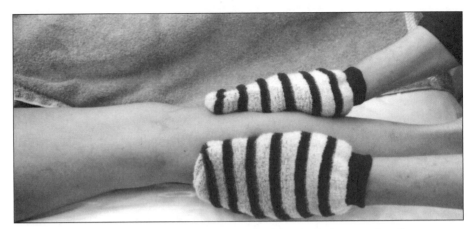

FIGURE 10-2 *Cover your hands with abrasive gloves and dry brush the area. This will stimulate circulation.*

(If using bed warmer in dry room, be sure it has been on prior to arrival of client.) If shower is not available, be sure to use a disinfectant or cleanser to preclean the body. If working on wet table, be sure client is properly covered with bath sheets or towels.

2. On a dry body, perform about 10 minutes of dry brushing on the front and back side (avoid all delicate and sensitive areas) to stimulate blood circulation (Figure 10-2). Use dry brushes, mitts, or massage gloves and move smoothly but fairly rapidly. This is the opening to the treatment so it should not be a massage.

3. Perform any special cleansing or exfoliation if applicable to the treatment (Figure 10-3) and rinse off well. If an exfoliant is used, skip dry brushing step. Client may shower off the exfoliant, or technician may wash it off. If washing off, remove plastic sheet. Below plastic sheet being removed another plastic sheet should be set.

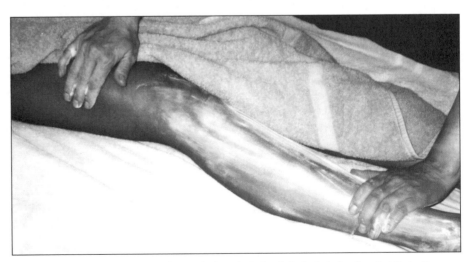

FIGURE 10-3 *An exfoliating scrub is applied to the body. If the body is dry brushed first, skip this step.*

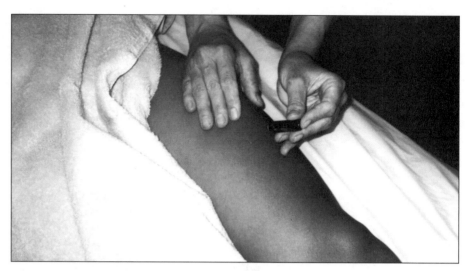

FIGURE 10-4 *Massage any aromatherapy oil into the body.*

4. Apply essential oils, treatment ampoules, or serums according to the goal of the treatment and massage into applicable area (Figure 10-4). This step should take no more than about 10 minutes. Cover client and allow product to absorb while preparing for the mud mask.

5. The application temperature of the mud may vary according to the manufacturer but is most often between 110 and 120 degrees F maximum. Be sure the temperature feels comfortable to the client. Mud should have been warmed in a double boiler, not a microwave. Use one hand only to apply the mud in a smooth even layer on one leg and one side of body (have client lie on side).

    Cover with plastic with free hand as you work up the body and then proceed to apply mud to the other side of the body wrapping the plastic as you go (Figures 10-5, 10-6). The final application will be to the front side

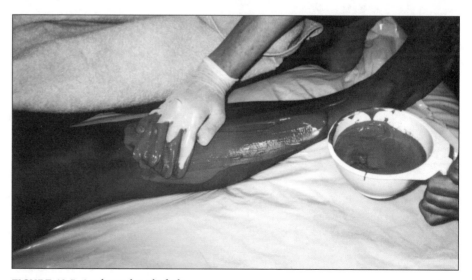

FIGURE 10-5 *Apply mud to the body.*

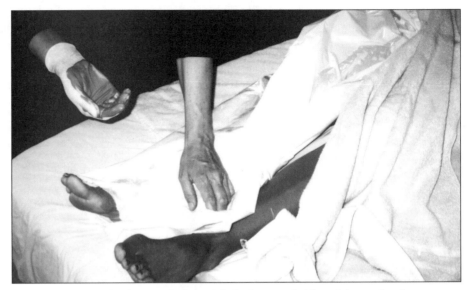

FIGURE 10-6 *Immediately wrap the body with plastic as you finish applying mud to the area.*

of the body. According to your treatment goal and client's comfort, you may apply mud on the stomach, chest, bust (except nipples), and neck area (Figure 10-7). If the client is shy and uncomfortable, skip the front except the décolleté area. After carefully wrapping the entire body in plastic, fold the sheet around and lay a bath sheet over the entire front (Figure 10-8). The client will rest about 15–25 minutes in the wrap.

NOTE: *Some muds are applied without plastic wrapping. If so, cover body with plastic or sheets and towels to keep warm.*

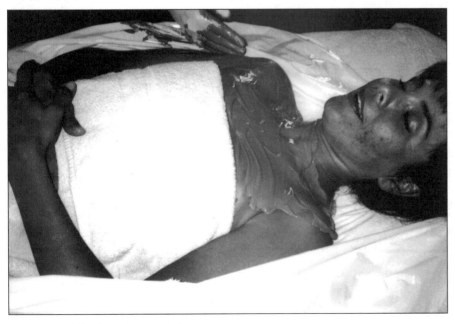

FIGURE 10-7 *Apply mud to the chest.*

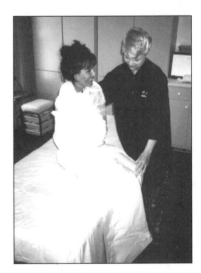

FIGURE 10-8 *Once the mud has been applied to appropriate areas and the body covered with plastic, wrap the client in a sheet. The client should rest for about 15–25 minutes.*

6. If you have a Vichy shower, open the sheets and let the Vichy shower rain comfortable warm water on the client's front side for 10 minutes, then 10 minutes on the back. You will need to get the client up off the bed for a quick spray shower to remove the remaining residue of the mask. If a Vichy or regular shower is not available, you will need to wash the client off with hot towels or shammies. Be sure the mask doesn't dry hard as it is more difficult and time consuming to remove. Also, allow the client to rest in the wrap 15 minutes to allow enough time for hand removal.

7. Put a fresh dry bath sheet on the bed and have the client lie back down facing up. Cover client with another bath sheet. Apply finishing body lotion or cream to the entire body. Apply finishing powder and help the client up and out to the rest area. While the client is resting, have her drink water or juice and discuss future treatment plans and home care program.

CONTRAINDICATIONS FOR TREATMENT
Do not use on clients who

- have high blood pressure.

- are pregnant.

- have active systemic disease or illness.

- have known allergies to components of clay, or iodine in cases of sea mud.

- indicate any questionable situation.

Summary of Treatment
1. Preparation of client.

2. Dry brush.

3. Special cleanse or exfoliation. If exfoliating, skip dry brush.

4. Apply special treatment oils, ampoules, serums.

5. Apply warmed mud, wrap, and let client rest.

6. Vichy shower and/or removal.

7. Fresh bed, application of cream/lotion, finishing powder.

Skin Cleansing Back Treatment

This treatment must use a mud designed to cleanse and draw out impurities. A soft moisturizing clay should not be used in this case. The treatment can be a short 30–45 minutes or 1 hour if full massage is being done. This is an ideal treatment for the client whose back breaks out.

GOAL OF TREATMENT
The treatment is normally very relaxing and stress relieving for the client, which indirectly may help the cause of the breakouts. However, the main

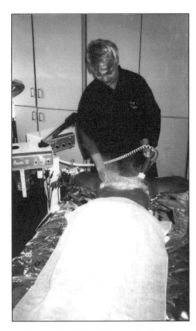

FIGURE 10-9 *Precleanse the back.*

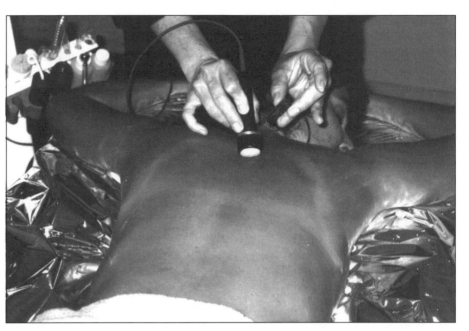

FIGURE 10-10 *Use the galvanic current for disincrustation cleansing on the back.*

goal of this treatment is to utilize the drawing out and purifying effects of the mud to clear the breakout area. If the mud is highly active, multiple treatments in a week may be necessary to draw impacted materials out. The treatment may be done twice a week until the area has cleared and periodically thereafter to maintain.

PROCEDURE

1. Prepare the client by having her/him wear a smock or remove upper body clothes, or completely undress as desired. Client should lie face down on properly draped bed. If bed has breathing hole, be sure to line hole with towel or disposable cloth.

2. Turn on steamer or warm back with hot towels. Precleanse with oily skin cleanser, deep pore cleanser, or washable cleanser (Figure 10-9). While steam is on, brush cleanse as desired.

3. Exfoliate as desired and/or apply disincrustant solution (Figure 10-10). Use negative galvanic current for disincrustation cleansing. (Be sure client can have galvanic done.) Rinse and soften skin with steam or hot towels or shammies.

4. Perform extractions of pustules and comedones (Figure 10-11).

5. Disinfect area with appropriate solution and high-frequency (direct) current (Figure 10-12).

6. Apply special treatment ampoule or serum if applicable, then massage with appropriate nutritional or massage cream (Figure 10-13). Massage time will vary according to the scheduling of the treatment. If doing a full-hour treatment, the massage can be 15-20 minutes long. If half-hour,

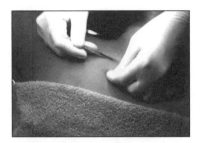

FIGURE 10-11 *Looking through a magnifying lamp, perform extractions of pustules and comedones.*

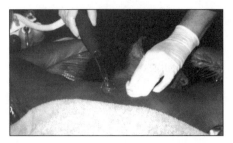

FIGURE 10-12 *Use the high-frequency current and an appropriate solution to disinfect the area.*

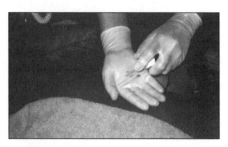

FIGURE 10-13 *Apply aromatherapy oils.*

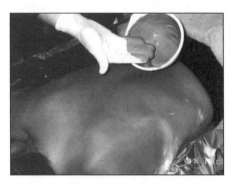

FIGURE 10-14 *Warm mud in a plastic container; apply liberally to the back.*

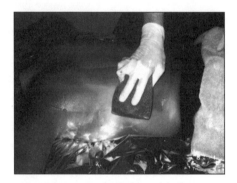

FIGURE 10-15 *Remove the mud with a sponge and warm water.*

the massage will last only 5–10 minutes at most. Use caution in massage if nodules and cysts are present.

7. Apply a thick layer of warmed mud to the entire back (Figure 10-14). Cover with plastic and then sheet and towels. Allow client to rest about 15–20 minutes.

8. Use hot towels or shammies and sponges to remove mud (Figure 10-15). Rinse well.

9. Apply cream/lotion and finishing powder.

CONTRAINDICATIONS FOR TREATMENT
Contraindications are the same as for full-body treatment.

Spa Manicure/Pedicure

Seaweed or mud can be used interchangeably in spa manicure/pedicures. If the goal of the treatment is to soften and moisturize the skin, muds in general may be preferable. If the goal is to relieve stress or swelling, seaweed may be a better choice. From the psychological standpoint, particularly if you're using manicures and pedicures to introduce your client to the body and spa department, then mud is the better choice. This may vary according to the manufacturer of your product line. Treatment should take 1 hour if full manicure/pedicure and polish is being done, 30 minutes if just treatment.

GOAL OF TREATMENT

This treatment will soften and condition the cuticles and skin as well as nourish and strengthen the nail bed. Follow-up home care with cuticle and nail strengthening cream as well as hand/body lotions and creams.

NOTE: *In this treatment, when hand/foot is mentioned, it includes arm and leg.*

PROCEDURE

1. Cleanse and disinfect hands and feet.

2. While one hand/foot is soaking, exfoliate the other. (If using foot bath be sure mud won't clog unit. Also other additives may be added to water as desired.) (Figure 10-16)

3. Massage one hand/foot with appropriate oil/serum/cream (Figure 10-17). Massage the other hand/foot. If product is treatment oriented, you may leave on residue and apply the mud over it.

4. Apply a thick coat of warmed mud and wrap hands/feet in plastic. (If you want the mud to stay warm and soft, put hands and feet in plastic liners and then put in electric mittens and booties. If doing both at the same time, you will need to allow the hands and feet to sit about 10 minutes.) While hands and feet are wrapped, the finger and toe nails may be prepared for polish application. Let mask sit for 10 minutes before rinsing. Be sure all traces of oil and mud have been removed.

5. Massage in hand/body lotion/cream while avoiding nails. Be sure nails are clean and dry.

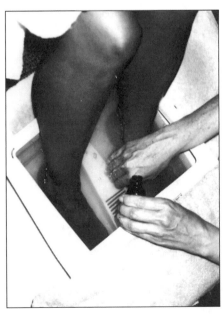

FIGURE 10-16 *Aromatherapy essences can be added to the bath water during pedicures.*

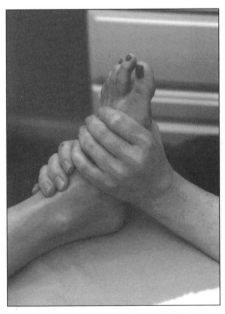

FIGURE 10-17 *Massage the foot, working the top and the ball of the foot.*

6. Apply polish as usual.

CONTRAINDICATIONS FOR TREATMENT
- Edema, infection, inflammation.

- Nail area if cleansing completely can't be done or mud stains.

Scalp Treatment

Scalp treatment may also be done with seaweed masks but depending on the scalp condition, a variety of muds may have more effects. In cases of excessively oily scalp, a drawing cleansing mud is ideal; where moisture and conditioning is desired, a nutritional mud is preferable. As in all scalp treatments, application and care of hair is important but most activity should concentrate on the scalp level. Duration of treatment is 30 minutes.

GOAL OF TREATMENT
Scalp treatments go in and out of style, but the need for extra scalp conditioning never leaves. The goal of this treatment is to stimulate the scalp circulation, moisturize, and soften. Dandruff may be alleviated by this treatment if done weekly.

PROCEDURE
1. Client's clothes should be protected by draping. If a hair steamer is available, turn on steam. If not, warm, relax, and soften scalp with hot towels/shammies. Use two or three and rub scalp slightly while towelling (Figure 10-18).

2. Apply massage oil/cream and perform about a 10-minute scalp massage (Figure 10-19). The length of time depends on the overall length of treatment. Leave oil or nutritional treatment on scalp.

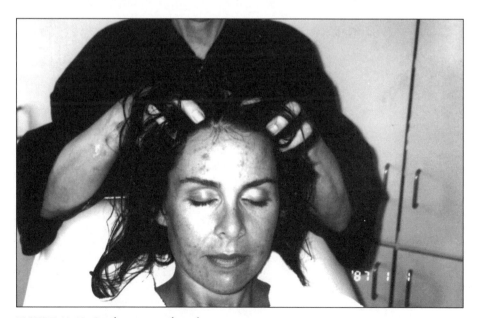

FIGURE 10-18 *Gently massage the scalp.*

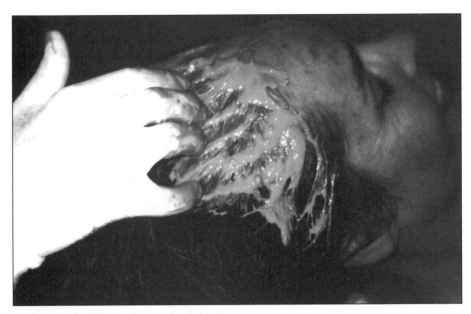

FIGURE 10-19 *With gloved hands, apply the massage cream.*

3. Apply warmed mud thickly to the scalp first and then to entire head surface. Wrap hair up into foil. Let sit 10–15 minutes. If you desire to keep mud warm, use heat lamp instead of foil. From time to time, check to be sure mixture is still wet and supple.

4. To remove, rinse hair from scalp out to ends, shampoo once or twice if necessary, and apply conditioner. Towel dry and proceed with styling. Do not do scalp treatments on same day as other chemical work (perms and colors). If possible, do chemical work prior to the mud scalp treatment unless as recommended by manufacturer.

CONTRAINDICATIONS FOR TREATMENT
Any type of lesions, open wounds, inflammation, or systemic disease.

• •

SPA POINT
Mud works effectively in full-body as well as spot treatments like hand and foot treatment, scalp treatment, etc. Mud will help mineralize the area, soften and recondition the skin, and in some cases draw out unwanted impurities, depending on the types of clay used.

• •

Mud Baths

Mud baths are certainly the psychological highlight of mud usage in health and beauty treatments. There are spas around the world that utilize natural hot thermal mud springs. The client is placed in the mud and covered for anywhere from 15 minutes to an hour depending on the thermal activity of the mud and health of the client. Some natural baths are constructed by laying the client on a bed of dirt that has been cut out about 3–5 inches deep and pouring warm mud over the body. The style is a little different but the goal is the same.

Most mud baths in America are traditional bathtubs or hydrotherapy tubs where 6–16 ounces of wet mud are added to the bath water for a hydrotherapy mud treatment. If the mud is sea mud, this may also be classified as thalassotherapy. However, utilizing the word *mud* is a more effective marketing concept. When giving a mud bath in this form, be sure that the type of mud you're using doesn't clog the tub. There are muds that will work well and muds that are too thick. Since mud holds its own heat well, use caution in putting too much mud in the tub or leaving the client in the tub too long. Follow manufacturer's instructions. Again, clients with high blood pressure or who are pregnant are contraindicated for this treatment. The tub treatment should last no more than 20–30 minutes. If mud baths are new to the client, it's better to leave the client in the water only 15 minutes.

Other Spot Treatments

Although some muds may be designed for bust, cellulite, and other spot treatments, as a general rule seaweed is more suited for these treatments because of its additives. If, however, your client is allergic to seaweed, a soil-based mud may be a good alternative. Be sure to understand what the specific mud is designed to do and then determine which treatments can be done with it. See also chapter 11.

USAGE OF MUD IN FACIALS

Almost all masks for oily skin incorporate either kaolin or bentonite and have for years. There are also softening masks for moisture. Recent scientific developments show greater promise for clays beyond their ability to draw impurities out of the skin or moisturize. The options are great and the formulations are vast. Some clays are even used now in massage and treatment creams, as well as in sunscreening formulations. Choose according to the purpose and skin type you're working on. Some people think a clay-based mask is old-fashioned. Quite the contrary. The opportunities for variation continue to grow and develop.

Synopsis

Mud has extraordinary cleansing and moisturizing/softening properties depending on the kind used. In this respect, mud offers a little more versatility of usage. From a marketing standpoint, mud is, of course, the most popular for spa conceptualization. The blend of mud and seaweed when appropriate makes for a multipurpose treatment system. Many exciting new muds are on the market, and the field will continue to grow. Mud was here thousands of years ago and will be here for many more. The time to use mud in full facial and body services is now.

Review

1. With what is mud synonymous?

2. Can clay be used on clients with high blood pressure?

3. For what is kaolin used?

4. Name two uses of clay in esthetics.

5. Should clay be mixed in a metal bowl?

6. Which type of shower is good for mud treatments?

7. Name one contraindication of mud treatment.

CHAPTER 11
Seaweed Treatments

OVERVIEW

Seaweed, an incredibly valuable source for effective face and body treatments, is a wondrous material you should know more about. Seaweed is a part of the greater family of life-giving substances known as algae. Alga grows in many places and as a result is a valuable source of material for cosmetic purposes. It grows in the sea, in lakes and ponds, in streams and rivers, in the soil, under ice and snow, and in the digestive tracts of human beings. We will concentrate mostly on sources from the sea, but keep in mind its existence in nearly everything natural, which makes it a valuable tool for the esthetician, massage therapist, nail technician, and hairdresser.

THE SEA

Of the 197,000,000 square miles of surface area on the earth, the oceans represent 139,000,000 square miles. Rivers and streams represent only about 1,000,000 square miles. In simpler terms, more than 70 percent of the earth is water. Water is not only the source of life for thousands of animal forms, it is also necessary for human life. Besides being essential from a drinking standpoint, almost 90 percent of the oxygen produced emanates from the plant kingdom, a large representation of that being from the algae that grow in the sea. Each gallon of seawater has approximately 1.6 cubic inches of oxygen, as opposed to 1.3 cubic inches in fresh water.

Seawater contains thirty-two to sixty different minerals and elements, including oxygen, chlorine, bromine, sulfur, sodium, magnesium, calcium, potassium, and silicon. Sodium represents about 31 percent of the seawater content. In some areas of the world, such as in the Dead Sea, the sodium content is much higher, which accounts for the tremendous buoyancy in that water. Seawater is also alkaline in nature. The sea is so rich in vitamins, minerals, salts, and proteins that it is purported to be able to support and feed all forms of plant, animal, and human life.

It has been said that human's blood plasma is so similar to ocean water that we evolved originally from the sea. René Quinton, a French biologist, wrote in his book, *La Mer, Milieu Organique*, that the human body originated in the sea and perpetuates the characteristics of its marine environment. He believed that the composition of blood plasma and concentration of mineral salts, proteins, and trace elements were so close that he transfused a dog's blood plasma with seawater and the dog survived; this convinced his colleagues. Truth or fiction aside, it is important to know that humans can benefit greatly from the sea. Seawater has been used for a long time as a natural remedy for sore throats, digestive problems, arthritis, and joint ailments.

ALGAE

Algae are plants that normally grow and thrive in seawater or fresh water, at the edge of water, and on some trees and rocks. In the ocean they often appear as undulating forests of slippery strands of grasslike materials (Figure 11-1). Algae are not grasses but appear in much wider ranges than almost any other plant group found on earth. There are more than 25,000 different known species, and their size can range from as small as a micron where more than 200,000 can lie on your thumbnail to as large as 200 feet long. Most of the common kelp used in cosmetics and other industries come from a large brown alga that commonly grows to over 100 feet. Most of the algae are beneficial to humankind, but some produce oily substances that are noxious, which give the water that marshy kind of smell, or at worst can be toxic and harm our fresh water and animal sources. Understanding algae completely is a lifelong process for many scientists.

It is interesting to note how algae function. Sunlight supplies energy that is absorbed by the chlorophyll in the algae. Carbon dioxide unites with the water forming a solid (sugars) and oxygen. The split off of hydrogen from the water molecule causes the sugars to form. In addition to the oxygen, the sugars convert to proteins from mineral salts containing nitrogen, sulfur, and sometimes phosphorus. Without these elements, the plant dies. Algae will

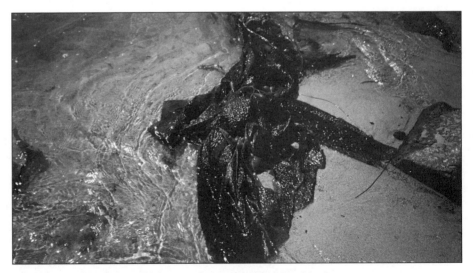

FIGURE 11-1 *Algae grow and thrive at the edge of seawater and fresh water.*

die in an aquarium where distilled water has been used. The conversion process from the sunlight is called photosynthesis. Thus the prime requisites for the growth of algae besides water are suitable light and temperature, carbon dioxide, oxygen, and mineral salts. The result is food for both plants and animals. Living creatures use the food, grow, multiply, and die; thus the food chain is perpetuated. The interesting thing about the growth of algae that makes them such a great resource is the fact that some (depending on the species) can grow up to 50 feet a day under the right living conditions. The growth of algae is closely connected to the amount of light received. That's why most algae grow in less than 200 feet of water. Due to the variety of species, some grow better in more light and some better in less light.

Chlorophyll is critical to the process of photosynthesis and algae are rich in chlorophyll. Algae are usually classified according to color. The name of the Red Sea comes from the abundance of red algae.

• •

SPA POINT

There are more than 25,000 types of algae, only a few of which are used in cosmetics. These are normally classified in groups according to color.

• •

Pigments in Algae

There are four basic pigments that comprise algae. Certain colors of algae are now being used as natural pigments for foods and cosmetics. As a pigment, algae use will see much future growth.

Chlorophylls (A,B,C,D,E):	Green
Carotenes:	Orange
Xanthophylls:	Yellow
Phycobilins:	Phycocyanin (blue)
	Phycoerytherin (red)

The location, temperature of the water, and sunlight exposure have a large effect on which algae grow where. Along with color, algae have been further categorized into certain zones.

FOUR MAIN DIVISIONS OF ALGAE
1. Chlorophyta: Green
2. Cyanophyta: Blue-green
3. Phaeophyta: Brown
4. Rhodophyta: Red

NOTE: *Other members of the algae group are categorized by silica—diatoms, stoneworts, etc. Diatomaceous earth comes from diatoms, or fossil algae.*

The economic value and importance of algae cannot be underestimated. The mere fact that some seaweed grows at exceedingly rapid rates makes it a wonderful renewable source for human use. Of course, the Chinese, Japanese, and Hawaiians have used various seaweeds for hundreds of years for food. In fact, the Japanese consume more than one hundred different varieties and specifically grow the algae for that purpose. Between World War I and World War II Japan was the only source of raw material supplies of seaweed for agar (solidifying factor used in laboratory culture) worldwide. It was the modern Japanese who first discovered uses for algae in mucilage for glue. Now the United States, Russia, Australia, and other countries are manufacturing sources for seaweeds.

The browns and reds are most often used in the cosmetic and food industries. Blue-greens are perhaps the oldest in history, and the greens provide the richest color and chlorophyll concentration. Some of the better-known species and economic uses follow. In cosmetics and body treatments, different varieties may be combined to enhance the mineral content, feel, or esthetic appearance. All algae, however, have value in cosmetics from a mineralization standpoint.

Seaweeds are rich in vitamins A and E and in inorganic salts such as iodine, which makes them valuable in glandular treatment and in laxatives. Specific uses and treatments will be discussed later in the chapter.

CHLOROPHYTA—GREEN
This division has a beneficial effect on skin firmness, improves circulation, and aids in moisturization and cell renewal. It is considered to be the most universally distributed in fresh and seawater. Lichen moss contains green algae.

Ulva: sea lettuce, often eaten as a vegetable

Acetabularia: umbrella-like

Halimeda: calcified

CYANOPHYTA—BLUE-GREEN
This division is high in vitamins A, B, C, D, E to stimulate metabolism. It is highly gelatinous, has a unique ability for fatty acid synthesis, and, due to a high quantity of chlorophyll A, it's highly responsible for molecular oxygen. Blue-green algae grow well in a hot springs mineral environment. They also grow in rice fields and may be a catalyst for increased rice growth. Lichen moss contains blue-green algae and they are found in the human digestive tract (duodenum, jejunum).

Calothrix

Rivularia

Nostoc: boiled and eaten with vegetables

Spirulina: highly valued for mineral content, used in food supplements, some cosmetics

PHAETOPHYTA—BROWN

This division is strong in metabolic stimulation, increases heat processes, helps in cellular exchanges and balances, and accelerates the elimination of toxins. It is most commonly used in foods, cosmetics, and industry and has high potassium and iodine content. Algin and alginate, produced primarily by laminaria, macrocystis, fucus, and ascophyllum nodosum, are used most often in foods, cosmetics, dental products, and fertilizers. Alkali salts can be spun into silk-like thread, and heavy salts form a type of plastic. This also forms natural gums so ideal in paints, car polishes, and pharmaceuticals.

Laminaria: often called sea kelp, used most often in foods (Japanese Kombu, Kobu, vast amounts grown in Japan), used also in medicine as possible coagulant and to help heal wounds

Macrocystis: largest sea kelp, may be the fastest growing plant known

Nereocystis: called sea otter's cabbage

Pelagophycus

Ascophylum Nodosum

Fucus: due to high iodine content, known to stimulate the thyroid

Sargassum: from Sargasso Sea, called gulfweed, rockweed, sea holly, used as thickener in soups and soy sauce

Chlorella: high in vitamin B_{12}, biotin, riboflavin, known to stimulate growth in chicken

NOTE: *The Sargasso Sea is an elliptical, very still tract of water in the North Atlantic Ocean. The Gulf Stream forms a portion of the western rim. The sea in this area reaches from 5,000 to 23,000 feet. Due to the weak air currents, low precipitation, and warm saline water, sargassum floats on the surface. It's kept at the surface by the small air bladders in the seaweed itself. This is a rich forest of brown seaweed. It was first introduced and discussed by Columbus in 1492.*

RHODOPHYTA—RED

This division mixes well with other species and serves as a stabilizer, filter, and lubricant. It is rich in iodine and very gelatinous. More than seventy-eight species produce agar, which is commonly used in jelly, as a soup thickener, as a clarifying agent in beer and other liquors, as a laxative and lubricant, and as the culturing medium in laboratory studies of microorganisms. Agar is used for preservation in canning fish, for sizing fabrics, for making film, for finishing leather, for adhesives, and in ice cream manufacture to prevent crystallization. Laver or Nori (Japanese term) is vitamin and mineral rich for food.

Chondrus: called Irish moss, produces carrageenin (an important stabilizer for cosmetic emulsions), agar-agar.

Corallina: a calcareous alga used in biological bone implants, may also be a good infrared filter

Rhodymenia: called dulse, used for food as a vegetable

Ceramium, Lithothamnium, Corallina, and Lithophyllum become encrusted with lime and help build up coral reefs. They are also used with diatoms in diatomaceous earth.

· ·

SPA POINT

The four basic algae color divisions do the following in spa treatments:

Green—skin firmness, increased circulation, moisturization

Brown—increases metabolism and heat, accelerates elimination of toxins

Blue-green—high in vitamins to stimulate metabolism

Red—as emulsifiers, balancers, and lubricants

· ·

Uses in Esthetics

In the field of esthetics and beauty, different mixtures and combinations of algae are used for a number of purposes, depending on the manufacturer, the product function, and the treatment concept. Some of these purposes include:

- High mineral content helps stimulate the body's metabolism and circulation. This increase in circulation facilitates the absorption of nutrients into the system and the elimination of toxins and wastes.

- The various mineral properties can soften and cleanse the skin, leaving the skin smooth, softened, and supple.

- The vitamins A and E as well as some of the mineral catalysts (such as selenium) serve as antiaging antioxidants. This helps skin cells function better.

- As small an amount as 3 percent has tremendous skin softening capabilities.

- Helps the body to better regulate itself.

- In hair products, algae are used as a softening and moisturizing agent due to the cationic charge. Increases hair bounce and body. With regular use, may help prevent hair loss.

- Cellulite consists of trapped toxins in the subcutaneous tissue. Algae help disrupt the fat cells by breaking the chemical bonds and allowing trapped waste materials to be released into the lymph system for subsequent removal. The trace minerals act as catalysts in normal enzyme reactions in the body to ensure normal metabolic releases. Among other agents, silicon in alga works directly on the proper utilization of nutrients and the subsequent elimination of toxins.

- Zinc, an important mineral in algae, is an essential biocatalyst in all endocrine systems. These systems have a direct effect on skin, so indirectly zinc will help stabilize skin. It is often used in acne treatments and as a sun protectant. Zinc is thought to help control excess sebaceous secretion.

- Magnesium and calcium are valuable substances as activators of other body systems, especially enzyme systems. Magnesium helps the proper metabolism of calcium, phosphorus, and sodium and is easily absorbed by the body. Calcium is integrally involved in the bones and intercellular protein cement. It has also been known to play a role in the permeability of the capillaries' blood coagulation and muscle and nerve stimulus. Magnesium is an important component of chlorophyll.

- Trace minerals may be bonded to proteins and be absorbed easily. The value of this in skin lies in the moisturizing ability of the combination above what is capable of the proteins alone.

- Because the trace minerals penetrate the body readily under good thermal conditions, they help rid the body of excess water and lipids and improve circulation. By doing so, a natural detoxification process takes place.

· ·

SPA POINT

As has been discussed in great detail, seaweed holds the key to a vast number of uses in today's world. As a cosmetic substance, we're only beginning to appreciate all that it potentially can do. With more scientific study, greater treatment development, we may soon discover that the riches of the ocean are our most potent and viable naturally renewing resource for modern day spa treatments and cosmetics. The varieties of seaweed do, of course, offer different practical applications. The reds and browns appear to be the most used at this point in time, but undoubtedly research will carry us to greater depths of appreciation and knowledge.

· ·

TREATMENTS IN ESTHETICS

General comments and treatments are presented for your information. Please be sure to obtain specific details and treatment procedures from your product manufacturers as systems and concepts, as well as types and amounts of seaweed, vary somewhat according to the manufacturer. Pricing for treatments should be made consistent with other services, market competition, and product cost.

Thalassotherapy Body Treatment

Thalassotherapy refers primarily to the use of seawater and seaweeds in baths and body treatments.

SUPPLIES NEEDED

Massage table or wet room table

1–2 cotton sheets (green or grey color due to staining of some seaweed)

3 bath sheets (or large bath towels, also green or grey)

2 hand towels

1 bathrobe

1 electric bed warmer if allowable

1 regular cotton blanket

1 plastic or foil sheet (foil preferred for heating treatment)

2–4 body shammies, or 2 large body sponges, or 4 hot towels (ideally kept in hot towel cabinet for ready warm moist usage)

1 pair dry brushes or mittens

1 large masking brush or spatula

1 large plastic or rubber bowl (stainless steel bowl for some usage is fine, but never have glass in treatment area in case of breakage)

1 large wooden spoon or whisk for mixing

1 set measuring cups and spoons

1 pitcher of cold water for client to drink (with cup)

EQUIPMENT NEEDED

Hot towel cabinet

Facial steamer

Hydrotherapy tub, showers

PRODUCTS NEEDED

Disinfectant

Cleansing products

Toning lotion/astringent

Essential oils/massage product

Alga powder mixture

Body cream/lotion (moisturizer, anticellulite, etc.)

Finishing powder

NOTE: Most seaweeds do stain to some degree, so choose linens and towels accordingly. Dark green is ideal when using green seaweeds as stains won't show. In some cases pure white stains the least. Check with your product manufacturer for recommendations.

Table Setup

Over table drape electric bed warmer, regular blanket, bath sheet, cotton sheet, plastic or foil sheet. Offer hand towel to client to cover breasts and have another hand towel as diaper if necessary. If salt or scrub exfoliation precedes seaweed treatment, put another plastic sheet over the first sheet. Keep in mind, foil is used when more thermal effect is desired. Use plastic only with heat-sensitive client. Whether the full body or partial body is done, the layering effect is about the same; just reduce size of foil and plastic as necessary.

Client Preparation

Preparation depends on the selected treatment. If a full-body treatment is to be performed, it is always preferable to have the client shower. It is also easier to perform body treatments if the client is completely nude and all coverage is provided by sheets and towels over areas not exposed for treatment. The need for a diaper and breast towel is determined individually by the technician and client. If the treatment being done is a local or spot treatment, that area must be exposed and precleansed.

SEAWEED TREATMENTS

Full-Body Seaweed Treatment

GOAL OF TREATMENT

The goal of this treatment can vary greatly according to the client's needs. If a specific need hasn't been determined, a general full-body seaweed treatment in a mask or wrap offers overall circulatory stimulation, encourages elimination of toxins, softens and smoothes skin, and gives an overall sense of well-being. The exfoliation and additives further enhance the skin smoothening and softening as well as facilitate the body's own systems. Obviously frequency of treatment further enhances the effects, and a series of four to six weekly treatments is ideal from a conditioning standpoint.

INDICATIONS FOR TREATMENT

All normal healthy individuals may receive treatments. Client must complete health history chart prior to treatment.

NOTE: The treatment procedures for spot treatments will normally follow a similar pattern as for the full-body mask or wrap. Variances normally occur in choice of treatment products and essential oils, amount of time left on the skin, and removal techniques. Therefore, the full-body treatment will be listed first.

PROCEDURE

1. Client should be placed on draped table after showering. Client should lie on back. Be sure client is immediately carefully covered and warm.

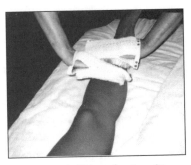

FIGURE 11-2 *Using abrasive mitts, stimulate circulation with dry brushing.*

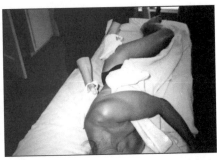

FIGURE 11-3 *Have the client roll onto the side and use abrasive mitts on the back.*

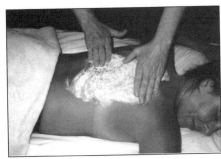

FIGURE 11-4 *Perform exfoliation on the back.*

(Bed warmer should have been on prior to arrival of client.) If shower is not available, be sure to use a disinfectant or cleanser to preclean the body.

2. On a dry body, perform about 10 minutes of dry brushing on front and back side to stimulate blood circulation. Use dry brushes, mitts, or massage gloves and move smoothly but fairly rapidly (Figures 11-2, 11-3). This is the opening to the treatment so it should not be a massage.

3. Perform any special cleansing or exfoliation if applicable to the treatment (Figure 11-4) and rinse off well. If an exfoliant is used, skip dry brushing step.

4. Apply essential oils or treatment ampoules according to the goal of the treatment and massage into applicable area (Figure 11-5). This step should take no more than 10 minutes.

5. Prepare the seaweed mask according to the manufacturer's recommendations. Normally 6 to 8 ounces of dry powdered seaweed is sufficient for the body. Mix with warm water. If essential oils are to be added to the paste, do so at this time and mix well (Figure 11-6). Apply mask with one hand only (clean hand is used to wrap the client in the foil or plastic) from the top of the feet, up the legs (Figure 11-7). Wrap the legs in the plastic or foil, turn client over to side and apply up the buttocks and back on one side and up the same arm and fold sheet over. Go to other

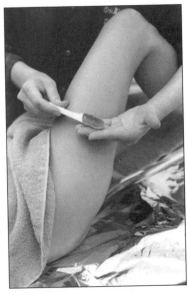

FIGURE 11-5 *Apply essential oils and massage into the area.*

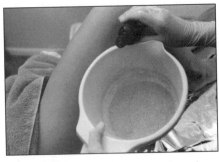

FIGURE 11-6 *Add aromatherapy oils to the pasty mixture.*

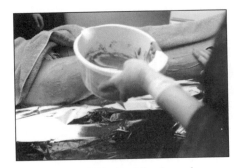

FIGURE 11-7 *With gloved hands, apply mixture to the body.*

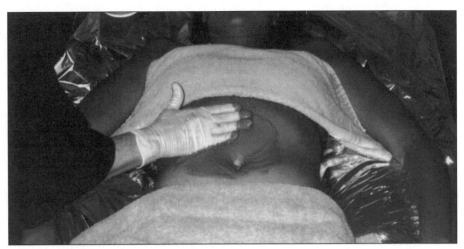
FIGURE 11-8 *Apply the mixture to the stomach.*

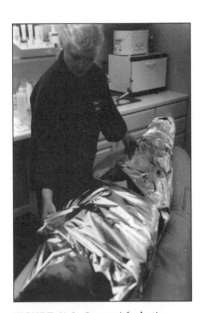
FIGURE 11-9 *Cover with plastic or foil.*

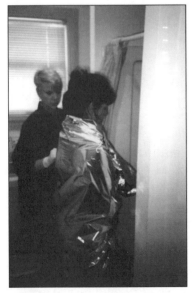
FIGURE 11-10 *Help client to the shower with the foil still loosely wrapped.*

side of bed, roll client on side and apply mask to backside and arm then wrap in plastic or foil. At this point client should be lying on back.

Be sure now that mixture is applied to stomach (Figure 11-8), chest, breasts (only if by permission), and neck and be sure plastic or foil has completely covered the body (Figure 11-9). Wrap the cotton sheet and blanket over the client in a snug manner. If the bed warmer is on, turn it off after 3–5 minutes to keep the client from overheating. This application method is called the "one-side, then-the-other-side method." Some prefer to have the client sit up to apply the mask to the back and then have the client lie back down and continue with the other procedure. Either method is fine as long as the client is comfortable and well covered as the application progresses. The application should normally be thinner than a facial mask but thick enough not to see too much skin through the mask. Massaging it on in circular movements not only feels good but helps the nutrients in the mask and oils applied under the mask or put into the mask absorb better. The client rests for 20–30 minutes. While the client rests, the technician should update the chart, determine the home care products and routines, and prepare for the mask removal. If the client becomes too warm during the treatment, the blanket and sheet may be unwrapped and pulled away easily leaving the client wrapped only in the plastic or foil. It's advisable to lightly cover the client with a towel.

6. If shower facilities are available, help the client get up with the foil or plastic still loosely wrapped (Figure 11-10). The client may discard the plastic or foil in the receptacle in the shower.

    If a shower is not available, use warm moist hot towels, shammies, or sponges and rinse the body off area by area starting at the legs and working up the body. As each area is cleaned, be sure to pull the plastic or foil out of the way. If the mask is still moist and is thick enough, sometimes a spatula or the palm of the hand is useful for removing the majority of the product and then you can just towel off the residue.

7. While the client is in the shower, place a fresh new bath sheet on the bed. When the client returns, apply moisturizing body lotion or cream and then finishing powder to complete the treatment. If removing by hand, finish entire removal and then apply moisturizing body lotion or cream and finish with the powder.

8. Help the client to sit up and rest for a moment before getting off the bed. Have the client rest in a chair for a few moments while you are explaining the effects of the treatment, future program, and the home care routine. This is the ideal time to consummate the sale.

CONTRAINDICATIONS FOR TREATMENT

*   Pregnancy

*   Any active disease or illness

*   Vascular problems such as high/low blood pressure

*   Known allergies to iodine or seaweed

*   Any questionable situation

Summary of Steps

1. Precleanse or shower.

2. Dry brush.

3. Special cleanse or exfoliation. If exfoliating, skip dry brush.

4. Massage in oils or ampoules.

5. Apply mask, let sit (put essential oils in mask if applicable).

6. Shower or wash off mixture.

7. Finish with body lotion/cream and powder.

Back Treatment

This treatment follows the basic full-body format with the addition of the disinfection with high frequency in step 5. Steps 4 and 5 will be skipped if extraction and disinfection aren't necessary.

This can be a short 30–45 minute treatment or a 1-hour treatment if massage is to be included. This is an ideal treatment for the oily, acne-prone skin, a male, or during the party season when women wear low or backless dresses.

GOAL OF TREATMENT

Generally the goal of most back treatments is to exfoliate skin that is difficult to reach on one's own. The back needs extra moisturization and softening as well. The back treatment provides a skin renewal that glows and feels great. If the client is acne prone, consistent back treatments on a weekly basis until the area is cleared is ideal.

PROCEDURE

1. Client can wear a smock, remove only upper body clothes, or be completely nude as desired. Client should lie on stomach on properly draped bed. If bed has cutout for breathing, be sure to line hole with disposables or washable towel.

2. Turn on steamer if available and begin to precleanse the back area with appropriate cleansing lotion or washable cleanser. While steam is on, you may choose to use brush machine to further cleanse area. (Options: dry brush, then cleanse; exfoliation on dry skin.)

3. Apply exfoliant or comedone softening solution (disincrustant solution and negative galvanic current for cleansing electrically; be sure client can have galvanic). Soften skin with hot towels and/or steam.

4. Perform extractions of pustules and comedones.

5. Disinfect area with appropriate solution and high-frequency (direct) current application.

6. Apply special treatment ampoule or serum if applicable then massage with appropriate massage product. Massage time varies according to the scheduling of the treatment. If doing a full-hour treatment, the massage can be 15–20 minutes long. If half-hour treatment, the massage will last about 5–10 minutes at most.

CAUTION: IF NODULES AND CYSTS EXIST DO NOT MASSAGE.

7. Mix about 1/2 cup seaweed mask mixture with warm water and add essential oils if desired. Application should be a little thicker than normal in order to allow the seaweed mask to absorb oils. Apply to the entire back and cover with plastic or foil, then cover with sheet, towel, and blanket to ensure warmth. Mask should remain for 15–20 minutes.

8. Use hot towels or shammies and sponges to remove mixture and rinse well.

9. Apply finishing lotion/cream and finishing powder.

CONTRAINDICATIONS FOR TREATMENT:

- Open wounds

- Sebaceous cysts or pustules

- Inflammation

Cellulite Treatment

It must be kept in mind that one cellulite treatment will show little if any effect. Cellulite is difficult, especially if it has been present for a long time and has evolved into "hard" cellulite. Hard cellulite has the characteristic orange-peel appearance, whereas soft cellulite shows less pronounced dimpling when the skin is pinched. It should be kept in mind that although seaweed is one of the best substances available to alleviate cellulitic conditions, the client must be consistent with professional treatment and home treatment and eating a high fiber diet, drinking tremendous amounts of water, massaging the area, and performing active exercise. Cellulite is not necessarily curable, but it is controllable. Cellulite is normally prevalent on women's thighs and hips and to a minor extent on the stomach and arm areas. Most men do not get cellulite. The treatment itself should be 30–40 minutes.

GOAL OF TREATMENT

This treatment is designed specifically to stimulate the blood circulation and metabolism in order to facilitate the body's expulsion of toxins. In simple terms, the stimulation charges up the metabolism and the fat deposits are prone to dissolving at a faster than normal rate. This is a progressive process and regular treatment once or twice a week for several weeks will show a progressive result. It's important to be using the proper follow-up products at home. Consistency and dedication are the key to success. Seaweed treatment for this condition is ideal.

PROCEDURE

1. Prepare the client as for the back treatment. The client may choose to change into a smock or expose the entire legs up to the panties.

2. Dry brush from the knees to the buttocks if other exfoliation is not being done (Figure 11-11).

3. Normally, a special cellulite product is applied directly to the skin. This product is often an essential-oil-based cream or gel and is designed to

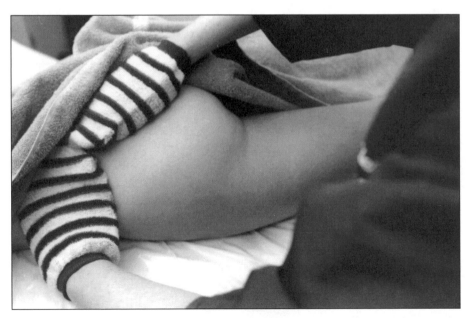

FIGURE 11-11 *Using abrasive gloves, dry brush the buttocks.*

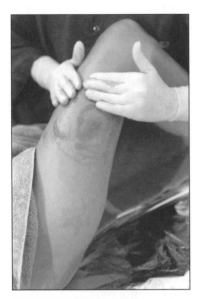

FIGURE 11-12 *Vigorously massage the cellulite product into the skin.*

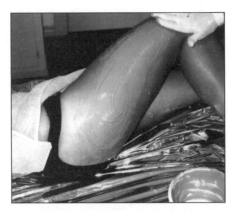

FIGURE 11-13 *Apply the seaweed mask to the thighs and buttocks.*

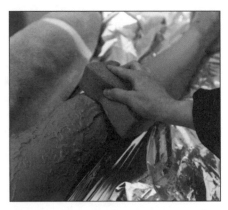

FIGURE 11-14 *Using a warm sponge, wash the mixture off the body.*

stimulate the circulation to the area being treated. This product is normally massaged in vigorously (Figure 11-12).

4. The seaweed mask is prepared with about 1/3 to 1/2 cup of seaweed with warm water and other additives as prescribed. It is then applied to the thighs and buttocks from the knee up (Figure 11-13). The area is then wrapped in foil or plastic. Foil is preferred due to the increased heat transference. The mixture sits for 15–20 minutes.

5. Wash the mixture off with hot towels, shammies, or sponges (Figure 11-14).

6. If the area has been reddened with a circulatory stimulant (vasodilator, which causes the capillaries to expand and causes redness), then it's advisable to apply a cooling solution or cream (vasoconstrictor, which soothes and causes the capillaries to contract).

7. Apply finishing lotion/cream and finishing powder.

CONTRAINDICATIONS FOR TREATMENTS

• Open wounds

• Varicose veins

• Bruising

• Sensitive skin

Localized Treatment for Achy/Sore Muscles

Different areas of the body can be treated in this manner—shoulders, lower back, arms, legs. The important thing to keep in mind with any spot treatment is whether to use a warming or cooling product under the mask. Where swelling may be present, cooling treatments are a must. Where parts of the musculature are just tense, warming treatments are ideal. In some cases, use of both warm and cool is invigorating and relaxing. Your product manufacturers will make specific recommendations on use. Keep in mind that when doing spot treatments it is prudent to do no more than two areas at a time.

GOAL OF TREATMENT

This treatment is designed to relax muscles and relieve stress and tenseness in the area.

CONTRAINDICATIONS FOR TREATMENT

- Broken bones
- Strained ligaments or tendons—avoid treatment without physician's direction.

Spa Manicure/ Pedicure Treatments

As sophisticated as this sounds, and as chargeable as it is, the actual procedure is quite simple. It entails following the regular manicure/pedicure procedure for the most part and then applying a seaweed mask mixture and wrapping in plastic during the time the other hand or foot is being prepared for polish. Also, depending on the type of seaweed used, the legs and feet can be rinsed off at the station in the footbath water. It's quite easy to use a hot towel or shammy to rinse off the hands and arms. The seaweed masking procedure must take place prior to application of polish, particularly if essential oils are involved in the massage or mask because they can dissolve polish. Special exfoliation also enhances the manicure and pedicure in a spa procedure. After removal of the mask, be sure to use a lotion/astringent to remove all traces of oils from the nails before polish application.

GOAL OF TREATMENT

The goal is to add a more advanced level of exfoliation and conditioning to the skin.

NOTE: *Where hand/foot is mentioned, it includes arm and leg.*

PROCEDURE

1. Cleanse and disinfect hands/feet.

2. While one hand/foot is soaking (if using foot bath, essential oils or special spa products including seaweed can also be added to bath water), exfoliate the other.

3. Massage one hand/foot with appropriate treatment oil, serum, or cream. Massage other hand/foot.

4. Mix about 1/3 cup seaweed mixture with warm water and essential oil additives if any and apply to each hand/foot and wrap in plastic or foil. While hand/foot is wrapped, prepare finger- and toenails for polish application. Let mask sit for 5–10 minutes. Rinse off and be sure all traces of oil have been removed.

5. Massage in hand/body lotion/cream on skin, avoiding nails.

6. Apply polish as usual.

CONTRAINDICATIONS FOR TREATMENT

- Open wounds

- Freshly shaved skin (legs)

- Inflammation

Bust Treatment

As shy as the American woman is, there is probably not a single female who wouldn't like her bustline to be in better condition. Bust treatments don't increase bust size, but they can work to firm, smooth skin, and soften the area. The manner in which bust treatments are done varies a great deal from manufacturer to manufacturer.

The following is a simple example. It is advisable to learn proper bust massage and check into legal limitations in your area prior to offering this service. Bust treatments are strong in Europe and their popularity is growing in America. Above all, keep the bust area covered as much as possible and keep movements firm. Prepare the client by having her wear a smock or removing her top. Cover the bust area with a large towel. Treatment duration is 30–45 minutes.

GOAL OF TREATMENT

This treatment is designed to condition and soften the skin on the breasts as well as to stimulate circulation to the area. The underlying pectoral muscles will also be stimulated to tone up.

PROCEDURE

1. Cleanse the bust area with a gentle cleanser, avoiding the nipples. Remove the residue with a warm shammy or sponges.

2. If an exfoliant is to be used, be sure it's very gentle and doesn't require too much rubbing. Avoid nipples.

3. Massage in appropriate massage oil/cream or treatment product for 5–10 minutes.

4. Prepare about 1/4 to 1/3 cup seaweed mixture with warm water and massage onto breasts avoiding nipples. Cover nipples with gauze or cotton pads and cover area with plastic or foil. Allow to sit 15–20 minutes. Do not allow mask to dry too hard.

5. Remove mask with warm water and shammy or sponges.

6. Apply finishing lotion/cream and finishing powder. Advise client of necessity of weekly or biweekly treatments and home care follow-up.

CONTRAINDICATIONS FOR TREATMENT

- Systemic disease

- Inflammation

- Bruising

- Tenderness to touch

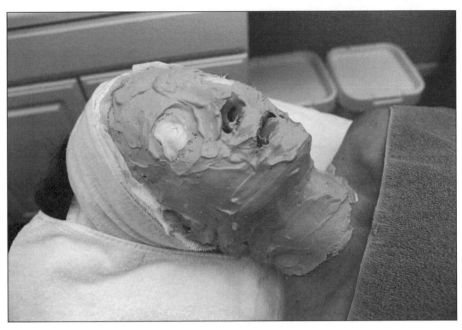

FIGURE 11-15 *Seaweed is a natural ingredient for facial masks.*

Facial Treatments

Naturally, seaweed can be used very effectively in facial masks and as additives to other systems (Figure 11-15). The most important thing to be cautious about when using seaweed in facial treatment is the potential for reaction. Seaweed is quite active and those persons with a potential for iodine or seaweed allergy responses can have severe reactions. It is always best to patch test before using in facial treatments.

· ·

SPA POINT

Seaweed is obviously great in all sorts of body treatments, from full body to cellulite. The types of algae may be different and can, therefore, perform any number of functions.

· ·

Thalassotherapy Bath Treatments

Spas and therapeutic treatment centers the world over use seaweed extensively in all water-related therapies. Seaweed can certainly soften and smooth skin, but its greatest benefit in a bath situation is the remineralization that takes place. As a rule, seaweed is micronized into a fine powder that when mixed with warm water converts to a highly absorbent state. Lying in a bath for 15–30 minutes provides phenomenal energizing and metabolic stimulation. As a bath additive, it's best to follow the manufacturer's recommendations, but in general add about 1 to 1-1/2 cups of seaweed to a quart of warm water and mix well. Then add to bath water when the tub is over half-filled. The skin will immediately feel smooth, soft, and conditioned. The metabolic improvement varies from person to person. But the treatment can be repeated daily to once a week if desired if the person is a normal healthy individual. See also chapter 3.

. . . .

SPA POINT

There is nothing more historical and effective than a thalassotherapy bath. This ideally combines the riches of hydrotherapy with the benefits of seaweed. Refer also to chapters 2 and 3 for full benefits.

. . . .

Synopsis

The results of using seaweed will be rapidly self-evident to the technician as well as the client. Seaweed provides myriad strategic benefits for the entire body or just specific parts and has been used since practically the beginning of time. With the development of scientific research methods and cosmetics, the future understanding of the value of seaweed on the human body will increase. Until then, seaweed as a natural invigorating source of skin and metabolic treatment should suffice. Unless there is a particular contraindication or allergy present, every client you see is an ideal candidate for this wonderful destressing substance.

Review

1. How much of the earth is water?
2. What is valuable for humans from seawater?
3. What are algae?
4. What are two main uses of algae in esthetics?
5. Name two specific body treatments with seaweed.
6. What is a common contraindication of seaweed usage?

CHAPTER 12
Other Treatments

OVERVIEW

"Other treatments" does not imply lesser importance than the specific treatments discussed under exfoliation, seaweed, or mud. The other treatments to be discussed here coincide with chapter 8 and will highlight the procedures for the spot treatments.

SPOT TREATMENTS

It's important to keep in mind that the various spot treatments can be done alone or in conjunction with full-body treatments. Coordinating all aspects may be a bit confusing at times, but the end result is a more effective treatment system and much greater profits. Also, different product lines will have different concepts and procedures so the procedures discussed will be generalized. You must refer to your manufacturer for specific step-by-step procedures.

NOTE: *All references to blanket in these procedures means that the bed will first have a bed warmer and then light cotton blanket. The bed warmer will be turned on prior to all treatments to keep the client warm and then be turned off during the mask waiting time. After mask removal it may be turned on again as needed to keep the client warm. Bed war not be used in wet rooms.*

Spa Manicure/ Pedicure

The spa manicure and pedicure will be similar to a normal manicure and pedicure except for the addition of a few steps and products. The next treatment, the hand and arm, foot and leg treatment, is also basically the same but without the actual nail care procedures. Understand that references to hand and foot mean arm and leg to elbow and knee as well.

GOAL OF TREATMENT
This is the ideal manicure and pedicure that adds a unique and client-holding dimension to normal nail care services without adding much time. Allow only about 15–30 minutes for the service. The spa addition will mineralize, exfoliate dead skin, and go far in extra softening and conditioning of the skin, cuticles, and nails. The mineralization is great for strengthening the nails.

PROCEDURE
1. Clean and disinfect client's hands and feet.

2. Starting with left hand/foot, remove old polish.

3. File nails of left hand and foot, then immerse hand and foot in hand and foot baths. You may add an aromatherapy bath gel or essence to the water if desired.

4. Repeat step 3 on right hand and foot.

5. While right hand and foot are bathing, the left hand and foot can be exfoliated. Use a salt mixture or body polish for this, not a dissolving enzyme due to the hand and foot soak softening the skin. Wash off salt mixture, push back cuticles with cuticle solvent, and clean under free edge of nails.

6. Repeat step 5 on right hand and foot.

7. Apply cuticle oil to cuticles and massage oil to hand and foot. Massage for 3–5 minutes. Repeat on other hand and foot.

8. Apply mud or seaweed mask on hands and feet and wrap in foil or plastic (Figure 12-1). If desired, a serum, lotion, or special treatment may be applied to skin before the mask. The mask will sit for 10–15 minutes and then be washed off. It's easy to wash the mask off the feet in the foot bath if the product doesn't clog the bath. Wash the hands and arms with hot towels, shammies, or sponges and dry.

9. Massage in finishing lotion or cream, but be sure there is no oil or seaweed residue on or under the nails. If necessary, use freshener to be sure all oil has been removed from the nails.

10. Apply base coat to nails and then two coats of polish. Apply top coat and spray with nail dry.

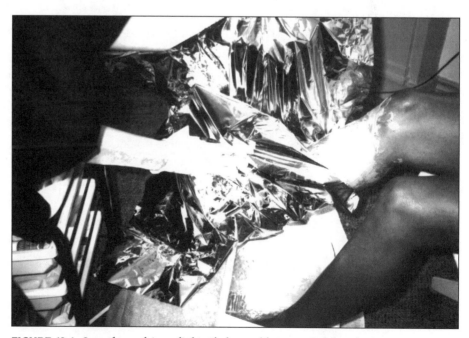

FIGURE 12-1 *Once the mask is applied to the legs and feet, wrap in foil or plastic.*

CONTRAINDICATIONS FOR TREATMENT

• Fungus or other nail disease

• Open cuts or wounds

• Edema, infection, inflammation

Spa Hand and Arm, Foot and Leg Treatment

As with the spa manicure and pedicure, the treatment should be done from the hands to above the elbow at least and from the foot to above the knee. These treatments are highly invigorating as was discussed in chapter 8. Either or both of these treatments may be incorporated with facial treatments, spot treatments, scalp treatments, or other hairstyling procedures. They also entice the consumer into returning for body treatments. When the technician has a little free time, it's good to offer a sampling of the effects of the treatment on one hand and arm just to show the client the difference. Obviously this means that your product and treatment must show a visible difference. Since the nails aren't being done, the hand or foot bath may be eliminated as desired. For the feet, it's nice to still use the foot bath. Again, the terminology will basically refer to the hands and feet but with the understanding that this includes the arms and legs.

GOAL OF TREATMENT

The goal of this treatment is to remove dead cells and soften, refresh, and condition the hands and feet.

PROCEDURE

1. Sanitize hands and feet with disinfectant spray. Technician's hands should also be sanitized or gloves worn as desired.

2. Cleanse the hands and feet with appropriate cleanser/toner.

3. Apply exfoliant and let sit appropriate amount of time. If the product requires mixing and a longer waiting time, you may want to apply product to one hand then the other, allowing you time to remove one while the other is processing. If it is a rub-off type product, you may rub off one hand or foot while the other one is waiting. If using the foot bath, you may also soak one foot in the bath while doing the other foot. Be sure to put some essential oil into the foot bath. You may also use a salt mixture for exfoliation for a spa effect. Be sure salt is not a problem for your foot bath.

4. If applicable, apply special conditioning or active solution. This may be a hydrating ampoule, a special aromatherapy lotion to stimulate circulation, or a menthol rub. Rub in well (Figure 12-2).

5. Apply appropriate massage product and perform a 5–10 minute massage.

6. Apply spa mask. This may be any number of masks but seaweed or mud will work best. Most muds that can be washed down drains will wash all legs and feet well in the foot bath with a sponge. Be sure to apply an

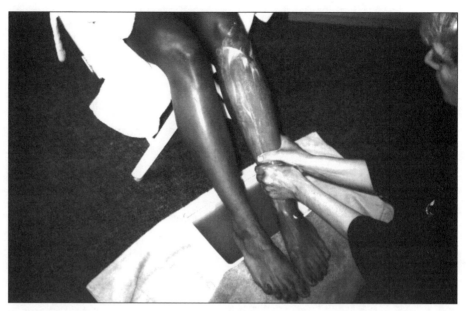

FIGURE 12-2 *An aromatherapy lotion can be applied to stimulate circulation.*

ample amount of oil or lotion around the nails of the hands and feet to alleviate the seaweed or mud collecting in those areas. A hand brush will still be needed to be sure the mud and seaweed comes off the nail bed. Another alternative to avoid the problem of mud and seaweed around the nails is to apply the product up to but not around the finger- or toetips. Wrap the hands and feet in plastic or foil as directed by the supplier. You should use smaller pieces of foil and plastic. Let the client rest for 10 minutes while you clean up and prepare for the finish. (Paraffin mask may also be done at this stage as an alternative.)

7. Remove the plastic or foil and wash off hands and feet. Use brush to be sure all traces of mud or seaweed are out from under the nails.

8. Finish with application of appropriate lotion or cream and dust feet with finishing powder (talcum powder will do also) to prevent the client from slipping.

CONTRAINDICATIONS FOR TREATMENT
• Fungus or nail disease

• Open cuts or wounds

• Edema, infection, inflammation

Scalp Treatment

Scalp treatments have been popular in years past and have recently experienced a resurgence in interest. Scalp treatments are wonderful in full-service day spas where hair is done. If you choose to do scalp treatments in a spa where no hair is done, the client must be informed that the hair will be washed but not styled. This is a very quick and viable treatment with or without other hair services.

GOAL OF TREATMENT

The goal of this treatment is to reduce head, neck, and scalp tension; relax the scalp's skin; condition and stimulate the scalp.

PROCEDURE

1. Shampoo hair and scalp.

2. Apply special treatment—conditioning solution, ampoule, or essential oil complex—and massage into the scalp area only, not hair.

3. Apply massage cream, oil, or hair conditioner and perform a 10-minute massage. The massage should include the neck and upper shoulders.

4. Apply mask. This may be seaweed, mud, or other appropriate spa-oriented mask. The head will now be wrapped in foil or plastic, then in a towel and allowed to sit for 5–10 minutes. If you have heat lamps or steam hair dryers, they may be used and the time shortened to 5–7 minutes.

5. Rinse the mask out and do another quick, light shampoo. Rinse, condition hair, and blow dry.

CONTRAINDICATIONS FOR TREATMENT

*   Scalp disease or open wounds

*   Overly sensitive scalp

*   Edema, infection, inflammation

Cellulite Treatment

The cellulite treatment is one of the most popular of all the spot treatments, and will be a great draw to your day spa. Although it has been said time and time again, it warrants repeating: cellulite is not curable nor is the treatment of it a weight-loss program. To have a viable effect on cellulite, the client must be willing to do the following:

*   Eat well concentrating on foods with a high fiber content and lots of fruit.

*   Drink lots of water (twelve to fourteen 8-ounce glasses a day).

*   Get active exercise.

*   Have the cellulitic areas massaged and stimulated by dry brushing or scrubs 2–3 times a week minimum.

*   Have appropriate in-spa treatments and follow home care product routines diligently.

GOAL OF TREATMENT

The goal of all cellulite treatments is to stimulate the circulation and metabolism to help the body eliminate toxins and wastes. It is also to help break up fat deposits that can in turn be flushed out of the body through the elimination system. A series of six to twelve biweekly treatments will offer the optimum results faster.

PROCEDURE

1. The bed will be set up as usual but with foil cut to fit waist to knee. If the cellulite treatment is being done with a full-body treatment, a full piece of foil should be placed on the bed. If exfoliation is being done as well, plastic should be placed on top of the foil. It will be removed after the exfoliant has been removed.

2. The areas of cellulite, usually from the knees to the waist including the backs of the thighs and buttocks, are normally treated. Cellulite treatments are also more effective if an exfoliation takes place first, unless there is quite a lot of varicosity. If you are not doing an exfoliation, be sure to dry brush the area first. If doing an exfoliation, apply the exfoliant of choice and massage well. This should be a fairly active massage to stimulate the circulation. After all the exfoliant has been taken off, remove the plastic from under the client.

3. Apply the cellulite treatment. This may be a gel, an ampoule, or an essential oil complex. Rub in well.

4. Immediately apply the mask. Do not do a massage at this point. The mask may be seaweed, mud, or whatever has been chosen. The client is immediately wrapped in the foil, sheet, and blanket and allowed to rest for 15–20 minutes. If doing a full-body treatment, the rest of the body would be masked and wrapped in the same foil. If doing full body, the waiting time is normally 30 minutes. The added 10 minutes on the cellulitic area is fine. (As a side note, this is a good time to start a facial, do an eye treatment, etc.)

5. When the foil is opened, it's important to shower immediately or wash the legs off well with hot towels to prevent the client from becoming chilled. The foil is then removed and the client should be lying on a clean dry towel. Ideally the mask will be showered off. If you have done a full-body wrap, the client stays mostly wrapped up to the shower and drops the foil in the shower. When the client emerges from the shower a new fresh dry towel and robe should be ready.

6. The finish varies from product line to product line, but since many cellulite treatments include products that stimulate the blood circulation through vasodilators (expands the capillaries), a vasoconstrictor (contracts the capillaries) should be applied if available. Then the treatment is completed with application of body lotion or cream. If doing the full-body, the cellulite spot treatment (vasoconstrictor) would be applied first and then the whole body would be finished with the lotion, cream, or designated product. Since massage wasn't done before the mask, a 30-minute or 1-hour massage is an ideal companion treatment. If massage is to be done, do not apply finishing lotion or cream. This will be covered by the massage product.

CONTRAINDICATIONS FOR TREATMENT

- Telangiectasia

- Hypersensitive skin

- Edema, infection, inflammation

Antistress Treatment

As stated in chapter 8, this is a term for areas of the body where muscles may be sore and achy, and where there may be a buildup of lactic acid. Treatments to relieve stress are very popular and should be done on a regular basis for optimum results. Antistress treatments may be done alone or in conjunction with another spot treatment and/or a full-body treatment. The procedure for this is similar to a cellulite treatment in most cases.

GOAL OF TREATMENT

The goal of this treatment is to relieve muscular tension, stress, and overall discomfort in the tense areas. Common areas for this treatment include the neck, shoulders, and lower back. It may also include knees and elbows. Sometimes this treatment is used after broken bone injuries. It should be done after all initial swelling has subsided, or only cooling treatment should be done. Physician consent should be obtained in advance.

PROCEDURE

1. The bed is set up with the blanket, sheet, towel, and foil. If exfoliation is being done, also lay down plastic. The size of the foil depends on the size of the area being done. More than one area can be done in one treatment as desired.

2. The area is dry brushed or exfoliated as appropriate.

3. The antistress product is applied. This will be an ampoule, essential oil complex, or lotion and is most often a vasodilator to stimulate the circulation.

4. The seaweed, mud, or other mask is applied and the client is wrapped in the foil, sheet, and blanket and allowed to rest 15–20 minutes. If it is being done in conjunction with a full-body treatment, the mask would be applied to the rest of the body then wrapped in the foil, sheet, and blanket and allowed to rest for 30 minutes. The additional 10 minutes is fine for the antistress portion.

5. The foil and product is then removed, preferably by showering if done on a full body. Remember, the client may chill when the foil is opened so it's best to help the client into the shower and let the foil drop to the floor in the shower. If only a small area was done for antistress, it's easy to wash this off with hot towels or sponges.

6. If a vasodilator has been used, a vasoconstrictor should be applied to the stressed area and then a finishing lotion or cream should be applied. Do not apply any cool product on the entire body. It can chill the client very quickly. Apply it only to the spot areas and then finish the

body with a lotion. Since massage hasn't been done with this treatment, a 30-minute or 1-hour massage can be a great companion treatment. If so, do not apply the finishing lotion or cream since the body will be massaged with oil or cream anyway.

CONTRAINDICATIONS FOR TREATMENT
- Edema, infection, inflammation.
- Broken bones. Obtain physician consent.

Bust Treatment

The bust area is a good treatment area for most women over thirty or pregnant women. Although the treatments should not be done on nursing mothers, it's an ideal pre- and posttreatment to help firm and tone the bust area. In many cases, due to the shyness of American women, the client should begin by using retail products at home and then expand to the spa once she has begun to get used to the idea. There is still hesitancy on the part of many women, but the desire for a better bustline is there. Do not make promises of increased or decreased size.

GOAL OF THE TREATMENT
The goal of all bust treatments is to stimulate the area to improve skin texture and feel and to help tone up the pectoral muscles and surrounding skin. The skin will have an improved firmness with a series of treatments. Bust and cellulite treatments require more frequent treatment and dedication to achieve the desired results. A series of six to twelve biweekly treatments is recommended. Bust treatments are also highly recommended after augmentation surgery to keep the area supple and implants soft and pliable. It's also great as a presurgical procedure.

NOTE: *The nipples will be avoided in all steps of the treatment and will be covered by tissues or cotton during the mask. All movements in the bust area should be hand over hand to reinforce the movements without jiggling the breasts. The movements should be firm. Figure eight and circular movements are recommended. The breasts should be kept covered as much as possible during the treatment. Depending on the product line and shyness of the client, most steps, including the massage, can be done by one hand with the other hand holding a towel over the area to avoid exposure of the breasts. This is normally not necessary after the client has experienced a few treatments but may be helpful in the beginning to protect modesty. Some treatments cannot do this at the mask stage due to clay or molding mask applications.*

PROCEDURE
1. The bed should be set up with blanket, sheet, towel, foil, and plastic if doing exfoliation. There should also be a hand towel to keep the breasts covered between steps.
2. Dry brushing is normally not done. A very light quick exfoliation is recommended. This can be included in the treatment without concern for too much added cost or time. Very little exfoliant is used and the procedure time is greatly shortened to just 1–2 minutes. The exfoliant is washed off with sponges or shammies and warm water. The breasts are covered.

3. There may be a large difference in treatment products. If it is a gel, you may want to put the gel in a small bowl and warm it before application to avoid chilling the breasts. Sometimes, the gel, ampoule, or substance is mixed with the massage cream and a 5–7 minute massage is performed. Sometimes vasodilators and vasoconstrictors are mixed to dilute the sensation for this delicate area, or the treatment products may be applied and then massage cream applied and massage done. The massage is normally done at this time rather than after mask removal, again for the comfort of the client.

4. The mask is now applied to the entire upper chest (décolleté) and breasts, making sure to avoid the nipples. The mask may be seaweed or mud. Only about 1/3 to 1/2 cup of the mixture will be needed unless otherwise directed. The nipples should then be covered with tissues, cotton, or gauze. The bust area is then wrapped or covered in the foil and allowed to rest for 15–20 minutes. Again full-body treatment or another spot treatment may be done at the same time. If so, after the mask has been applied to the bust area, the rest of the upper arms, chest, stomach (if applicable), and back should be covered and wrapped. Then finish the rest of the body. In some cases, technicians prefer to sit the client up, apply the mask on the back, lay the client back down, and then apply it to the chest and arms. The most important thing is to keep the breasts covered and protected at all times. Whichever method works best for you is fine. This procedure will also vary with different treatments. If full-body treatment is being done, the extra 10–15 minutes will not normally be a problem. But if it is, you may need to open the wrap, rinse the bust area, cover it with a dry hand towel, and rewrap for the remainder of the full-body treatment.

5. At removal, if full-body treatment is done, showering is the best. If only a bust treatment is done, the foil should be opened and the bust area washed off quickly with hot towels or shammies. The faster the better. Re-cover with towel.

6. If a vasodilator was used in the treatment, now apply a very small amount of the vasoconstrictor or dilute it with the vasodilator so the client doesn't chill. Apply a finishing lotion or cream and massage in well. Cover the breast area and finish the rest of the body if applicable.

CONTRAINDICATIONS FOR TREATMENT

- Lactating (nursing) mother

- Edema, infection, inflammation

- Immediately after surgical procedure; obtain physician consent

- Systemic disease such as breast cancer

Back Treatment

Of all the spot treatments available, this is probably the most desirable one. Many people will come in to try a back treatment even before a full-body treatment. Back treatments, or back facials as they are sometimes called, are immensely popular for women during the holidays and high social seasons due to backless evening gowns. For teenagers and many men, back treatments can help correct acne breakouts and infections. They are very stress relieving and relaxing.

GOAL OF TREATMENT

1. To deep cleanse an area difficult to reach in normal daily care

2. To exfoliate excessive dead cell buildup

3. To facilitate the expulsion of excess oils, removal of comedones and pustules

4. To moisturize and condition the back

5. To relax and reduce stress

6. To relieve muscular tension on the neck, shoulders, upper and lower back

PROCEDURE

1. The bed should be set up with blanket, sheet, towel, foil, and/or plastic. The client this time will be lying face down, so if you have a bed with a breathing hole or facial cradle be sure the area is lined with a towel or disposable paper covering.

2. The back is first cleansed or dry brushed. Cleansing and exfoliation are strongly recommended. After the area has been cleansed and rinsed with hot towels, the back should be ready for exfoliation.

3. Apply the chosen exfoliant and work into the back well. The back area can handle a little more aggressive treatment. Some technicians even like to use the electric brushes from the facial machine to deep cleanse the back. If appropriate, a steamer may be used in conjunction with the cleansing or exfoliation procedure.

4. After the removal of the exfoliant, the plastic underneath should be removed. Then manual extraction of comedones and pustules should take place if applicable. Immediately after extraction the area should be disinfected and high-frequency current may be used directly on the skin as long as there are no contraindications. The contraindications for back treatment will be the same as for any facial treatment. Gloves must be worn by the technician during the extraction and after if anything was extracted.

5. After the area has been disinfected, any special treatment products such as ampoules, lotions, serums, or essences may be applied. Then the massage is normally done for about 10–15 minutes, concentrating on areas of tension and stress.

6. The appropriate mask is then applied and the back wrapped up in the foil or plastic. The mask may be mud, seaweed, or any other product desired. Sometimes a clay-based mask is used to help draw out dirt and oils. Sometimes a combination of two masks is used. After the client is

wrapped and covered with the sheet and blanket, the resting time is 15–20 minutes. A full-body treatment can also be done in conjunction with a back treatment, but a back treatment is most often done alone.

7. The foil is then removed and the back either washed off or showered off. If washed off, hot towels are ideal and feel very relaxing to the client. The treatment ends with finishing lotion or cream and sometimes with a finishing powder to be sure no oil bleeds onto the clothes. Back treatments should be done weekly in a situation where the client is broken out. For anyone else, a monthly back treatment would be sufficient.

CONTRAINDICATIONS FOR TREATMENT
- Edema, infection, inflammation

- Any heart condition if high-frequency current is planned for disinfection

- If the person can't lie on the stomach for 30–45 minutes

Spa Facial

As stated in chapter 8, a spa facial is actually nothing unusual except for the use of more aromatherapy, seaweed, and mud. Some seaweeds and muds are designed for the face and some are not. Be sure to check with your suppliers before arbitrarily putting body products on the face.

GOAL OF TREATMENT
The goal of the treatment would be to take a regular facial and make it appear more spa-like by adding seaweed or mud with a concentration on marine extracts and aromatherapy. Although aromatherapy is often used in facials anyway, you may choose to create special aromatherapy massage and masks that are more similar to body treatments. How the treatment is done is up to the manufacturer, but for simplicity a sample treatment follows.

PROCEDURE
1. Set up facial bed by placing a blanket then sheet over the bed and folding it into a cocoon shape for the client to get inside of.

2. The head is wrapped in a towel and headband; a towel covers the chest area.

3. The eye makeup and lipstick are removed with cleanser first, then the face is cleansed. Cleanser is removed with sponges or a shammy, and a freshener is used to remove the residue.

4. A deep pore cleanse takes place under steam. (Sometimes the brush machine may be used for a mechanical cleansing.) Steaming continues for about 5–7 minutes and then the face is washed and rinsed until clean. In lieu of a deep pore cleanser, an exfoliant may be chosen at this point. The application and duration vary with the product, but normally take less than 5 minutes.

5. If extractions or galvanic disincrustation is to be done, it will be done now. Be sure to wear gloves for the extraction. If galvanic is being used, the treatment should be for disincrustation with the current on negative, and then positive to restore the pH balance or to penetrate a water-based ampoule or serum.

6. Immediately after the extraction, the areas of extraction should be disinfected and then high-frequency, direct current applied.

7. If a special ampoule or serum is to be used, it will now be applied, and then the massage takes place. This should be an aromatherapy massage of some kind for about 15 minutes.

8. A spa-like mask of mud, seaweed, or similar substance is then applied. The mask sits with or without steam for about 10–15 minutes and then is washed off.

9. The skin is toned with the freshener and day cream is applied to finish the treatment.

CONTRAINDICATIONS FOR TREATMENT

• No electrical equipment on client with pacemaker or heart condition

• Be cautious with high and low blood pressure or systemic disease

• Do not use electricity on a pregnant client

• Do not use substances of known allergies; be careful about iodine in seaweed as some are allergic to it

• Edema, infection, inflammation, telangiectasia

• Anytime in doubt

. . . .

SPA POINT

It's important to remember that all spot treatments can be combined in a multitude of ways. Many will be done in conjunction with hydrotherapy. For example, any usage of mud, whether just for a local area of for the whole body, rinses off well in a wet room environment, hence the Vichy shower is a great add-on. Any spot treatment done with seaweed or mud and a wrap is easily tied to a full-body treatment of the same or similar kind due to the application of the same substances, wrapping, etc. The name of the game is to combine for efficiency, to maximize treatment potential, and to generate more business and income in about the same amount of time.

. . . .

OTHER HOT AND COLD TREATMENTS

Hot and cold adds dimension to spa body treatments. We have already discussed them from a product and water standpoint but a few others should be briefly mentioned here as well. A point of quick review—heat is stimulating and relaxing; cold invigorates and soothes. Cold is used to calm redness and swelling. Heat is used to stimulate the circulation and metabolism. The following modalities help increase the effects of the treatment goals by using cold or heat.

Hot Treatments

SAUNA

This is a dry heat room with a temperature over 176 degrees F. The sauna originated in Finland and is used in combination with cold plunges in the lake or snow to contrast hot and cold treatment, similar to a Kneipp concept. People who don't do well in moist heat will do well with short interval sauna time. The ideal situation is to use the sauna to stimulate circulation and perspiration, and then to briskly cool off. However, one must be very careful if not accustomed to this. In that case, it's better to sit in a sauna for 5 minutes and then slowly cool off for a few minutes. With time the duration in the sauna and the degree of cold after the sauna can increase.

People who don't do well in a sauna should consider moist heat. Some asthmatics do better in a hydrotherapy tub than in a sauna. Saunas are popular in health clubs; therefore, if you're not purchasing all modalities, a sauna might be one to pass on in favor of the more versatile Vichy shower or hydrotherapy tub considering the mix with products and treatments.

PARAFFIN

Hot paraffin has been discussed briefly in other chapters. The overall purpose of paraffin is to form an occlusive mask over the skin to seal it off. The heat makes the skin perspire and the moisture combines with the oils in the paraffin or whatever has been applied and absorbs back into the skin. The heat from the paraffin also stimulates the circulation. Paraffin is a viable mask to use in almost all treatments—full body, hand and foot, cellulite, back, bust. Do not use paraffin in scalp treatments.

Paraffin is popular in winter as well. Gauze is dipped in the hot paraffin and molded to the skin of the client where the treatment is being applied. At least three to six layers are applied, and the area is wrapped or covered in plastic and then a towel to hold the heat as long as possible. Usually paraffin stays on about 10–15 minutes. Once it's lost the heat, it's not very beneficial. Parafango is paraffin with the inclusion of fango mud (Italian volcanic ash and sulfur) to increase the mineralization of the treatment.

Although people used to like to dip hands and feet directly into the paraffin, this is not very sanitary and is now prohibited by most states. Wrapping with gauze is the most sanitary method. Under no circumstances is the paraffin to be reused. Paraffin is a great mask, but do not use it over areas of telangiectasia, infection, inflammation, or on the face of a claustrophobic client.

THERMAL MOLDING MASKS

These are very exciting masks for people who are not claustrophobic. They are normally made of a combination of alginates. Once the powder is mixed with warm water, the technician normally has about 4–5 minutes to apply to the skin over gauze. As the water and skin temperature come in contact with the alginates, the mask begins to harden in a manner similar to plaster of Paris. The mask will normally warm and cool, warm and cool until completely hard. The hardened mask can be removed from the skin in one piece. These masks are available for the face as well as for spot body treatments, and some even for the full body. The major contraindication to these masks is telangiectasia, sensitive skin particularly to heat, and claustrophobia.

Cold Treatments

There are now masks that work in a manner similar to paraffin but due to the coldness are better for the client with sensitive skin. Sometimes cold will help a skin care product to absorb better than hot and without the irritation heat causes some skins. Cold is popular in the summer, for men, and also for sensitive skins. It's also nice to alternate hot and cold in the same treatment. Cold masks are made from a powder alginate complex that is mixed with ice water. It then cools and hardens into a rubber-like texture. When the cool effect has worn off the mask is no longer valid and can be removed.

• •

SPA POINT

Hot and cold mask treatments may be used seasonally for variety or in conjunction with each other. A paraffin mask can be followed by a cold mask to soothe any redness from the stimulation of the paraffin mask and to cool the skin down. Both penetrate well, and cold masks may be used sometimes where hot masks such as paraffin cannot.

• •

Synopsis

Spot and special treatments are vital to the success of the day spa. They should be demonstrated to clients and used as a draw for the bigger treatments. The ability to mix and combine several treatments at once makes this a highly profitable field when marketed well. See *Day Spa Operations* for more business ideas on marketing the services. But remember, the better they are marketed, the more successful your day spa will be.

And finally, to make the most of the spa treatments, treatments and products must be used at home. The next chapter will discuss this.

Review

1. Why are spot treatments good for the spa business?
2. Is a spa manicure/pedicure the same as a hand and foot treatment? If not, how is it different?
3. What are the main goals of a cellulite treatment?
4. For what is a back treatment good?
5. What constitutes a spa facial?
6. What is a sauna and how is it different from hydrotherapy?

CHAPTER 13
Home Care

OVERVIEW

This is the most important chapter in the whole book. The point is simple; a good home care program makes the day spa program successful. As I have said in classes for years, what good does it do to give a great facial or body treatment if the client goes home and washes her face and takes a bath in Tide detergent? We all laugh at this, but it is a true story that happened many years ago with a facial client. Technicians have no trouble acknowledging the necessity of a home care program in theory, but in reality they often never discuss home care with the client. As discussed at the beginning of this book, it's common for massage therapists to think only about massage and estheticians to worry so much about the face that body never comes up. The blazing reality that must be faced it that body care must be taught to your clients and encouraged on a regular basis.

Another issue that must be corrected is that body care is a necessity, not a luxury. It would be wise for you to eliminate words such as "luxury" and "pampering" from your brochures and treatment menus. As long as consumers are presented with these words, they will continue to think of body treatment as luxuries and pampering, both of which can be quite easily lived without. Even though a treatment may feel luxurious or pamper the senses, it should never be sold that way.

. . . .

SPA POINT

In a day spa environment, the menus, brochures, and terminology from the owners and technicians must all portray a view of body care as a necessity, not a luxury. Luxury connotes something you can readily live without. The day spa belief is that to have a more successful, healthful life, body care is not something you can live without. Rather, it's a serious, viable way to be the best you can be. This has to be taught to the consumer.

. . . .

BASIC BODY CARE NEEDS

Just as one must train a facial client to use cleansers and fresheners or a hair client to purchase professional shampoos instead of the grocery store versions, it's also essential to draw your clients away from the bar soaps they see advertised so wonderfully on television. From soap to what?, you may ask.

As may be seen in grocery, drug, and department stores and specialty body and bath shops, there are hundreds of versions of soap, from the inexpensive grocery store brands that dissolve almost as fast in the bathtub by themselves as when they're used, to the gorgeous colorful transparent bars seen in the specialty shops. There are also bubble baths, bath salts, bath beads and balls. What does this tell you? Yes, that the first and most important product for consumers is soap. Soap of some form is the number one selling product in all the stores we've named. So your goal must be to move your clients to purchasing their soaps from you. Your product line must have some type of soap, hopefully a better soap than most.

Soaps

BAR

There's nothing wrong with a bar of soap as long as it's a good one, is made with great ingredients, and moisturizes and cleanses without overstripping. Transparent soaps are often good because they are usually made with glycerin, which is a natural humectant. The other ingredients should be skin friendly as well. The bar soap users are generally kids, teenagers, men, and busy women. Historically Americans are bar soap users so if you have a good one, they're easy to sell, and if the ingredients have a good story, it will be easy to switch the clients to your product.

SHOWER GELS

Shower gels are very popular but are generally not for regular use. The product may not actually be a gel, but a lotion, but it is a liquid or creamy form of soap. Normally these products must also have high sudsing ability. People like to try new shower gels because of the way they look or smell, or because they feel excited for the moment. However, consistent repurchasing is weak because people often feel that too much is wasted in a wash cloth or drips out of the hands before reaching the body. In other words, because they can be perceived as expensively wasteful, sales are often sporadic at best. Your shower gel sales will mirror this trend unless you help clients save money.

The very best, perhaps only, way to sell shower gels is in conjunction with a big, porous, soft sponge that will hold the soap well so less shower gel is actually used at one time. This may seem to you like it makes the soap last too long, but in reality it doesn't. It makes it a practical, viable purchase. A client can wash the whole body (assuming the shower gel is good) using very little soap in the sponge; the soap lasts longer and the client is happy to repurchase. Always sell liquid soaps with a sponge as a set.

Who uses liquid soaps? Women, and particularly those with dry skin. Liquid soaps are perceived to be more moisturizing. Men are not normally typical buyers of liquid soaps. They would be, however, if the soap could double as a shaving cream. Most can't, but some can. This category of soap will grow in sales with the right presentation to the client. It's great to have both a bar of soap and a shower gel for variety. Use one in the morning and the other at night.

Bath Additives

BATH SALTS OR BUBBLE BATHS

Bath salts or bubble baths are traditionally the fun part of body care. Bath salts aren't even salt. Typical bubble baths that bubble well are merely detergents with pleasant colors and fragrances but at a higher price. In America, bubble baths and bathing with them is perceived as a fun way to get clean and relax at the same time, before a party, when depressed, or upon landing a new job. There is very little serious consciousness as yet. However, this is an area where the day spa concept will really shine and where you can begin to make great headway with your clients. But first you must teach clients that these products from your day spa are serious; they are baths for a purpose.

Most well-designed professional bath salts or bath additives are certainly designed to cleanse somewhat, but they are also designed for treatment purposes. Some aren't for cleansing at all but strictly for treatment. In combination with the benefits of bathing, the additives may work to stimulate the metabolism, help break up fat deposits in cases of cellulite, relax sore muscles, or tone up skin. A milk bath or a bath oil, for example, works to soften, condition, and soothe skin. Bath additives are often based on aromatherapy and/or seaweed and mud. Everything you have learned about both will help you sell and promote these products.

Bath additives should actually be considered a baby day spa treatment at home. And in fact, they are. But the point that has to be carried over is that they are seriously designed for regular use, not just hit and miss for fun, and that they are actually a viable therapy. For example, normally most men would never consider in a million years taking a bubble bath. But what if you offered a man working in a high-stress situation the opportunity to relieve stress, relax muscles, and tone up the skin by lying in a bath for 20 minutes. He could even read the *Wall Street Journal* if he wanted to. Do you understand the presentation here? You will not present bath additives as fun bubble baths. You will present them as treatment. And as such, you will control and recommend how and when the clients use them. This gives you ongoing input into your clients' home care programs. This category of product alone will help you take charge of your clients!

BODY SCRUBS

Of growing popularity, body scrubs follow in the footsteps of facial scrubs because of the increased awareness of the need to exfoliate dead skin. Body scrubs are presented in every shape, size, and format and are often a television highlight. Many people who don't want to spend the money on scrubs accomplish the same thing by purchasing loofahs, mitts, or abrasive cloths. The reality is that they really don't replace scrubs. Although this author doesn't recommend scrubs for the face a scrub on the body once or twice a week is great. The advantage of a scrub over a loofah, for example, lies in the fact that the loofah is only a raw abrasive with no buffering capability or moisturizing capacity. Most scrubs are at least in a cream that has some kind of emollient base to cut the immediate roughness of the abrasive granules.

The granular scrubs are made with a variety of scrubbing grains, from the pits of certain fruits to nuts, oatmeal, pumice, silicone, or polyethylene balls. There are many different textures of scrubs and the one your client should use is yours. Why? Because you know best how it should be used. Consumers can't receive proper advice on the strength of the scrub in a department- or grocery-store environment and may develop resulting problems with skin sensitivity or irritation. However, you know your scrub and you can give specific instruction on how best to use it beneficially without harm. This is a simple product that is well understood by the public. What they don't know is the negative skin sensitivity part and you can save them with this explanation alone. Who likes scrubs? Everyone, but particularly men, teenagers, and those with oily skin. Even though it isn't recommended for the face, people with oily skin delight in rubbing, scrubbing, and stripping their skin. They are instinctive buyers of this product. You will then have to keep them from using it on the face.

SPA POINT

Your line can and will sell to consumers because the body products you sell also exist in a similar format in grocery, drug, department, and specialty stores. But what makes you better able to sell them is your professional expertise on how to use them more efficiently, more effectively, and more economically. Soaps, scrubs, and bath additives are all essential products; just present them as such.

Body Conditioning and Moisturizing

Unless all your clients happen to be young and have perfect bodies, they can all use some form of moisturization after bathing and showering. As long as they have skin, they will need these products. Keep this in mind at the outset and your sales will automatically increase. Additionally, as with all products, professional ones are generally more intensive or concentrated and targeted to special needs.

BODY MILKS/LOTIONS

Usually body milks and lotions are in a liquidy milky emulsion designed for quick application and absorption. They generally are not overly rich in emollients and are, therefore, ideal for day-to-day all-purpose body care. Everyone needs a body lotion or milk after bathing and at bedtime. Women tend to like fragranced body lotions and men generally will gravitate to unscented versions. There can be a happy medium within many of the aromatherapy bath products available, light but natural and results-oriented scents.

When you sell any cleansing product, you should, in fact must, sell a moisturizer as well. A common deterrent for sales of body lotions is the ability of clients to purchase quite large sizes of Brand X in the grocery store for much less money. One answer to this is typically, "You get what you pay for." But a better approach might be to explain that general body lotions aren't really targeted for much more than adding some emolliency; cooking oil can do the same. However, professional products generally are concentrated in highly effective ingredients that do more. Additionally, being concentrated, a smaller amount often works better and in the end less product is used so the price to use value is offset. In other words, a very high quality concentrated lotion may last as long as a jug of Brand X because of the concentration and added effectiveness.

BODY CREAMS

Body creams may perform in the same manner as lotions but are much more concentrated and in a cream base that will have more emolliency. It won't absorb as readily as a lotion and is, therefore, targeted to the drier skins and drier climates. For example, you might be happy with a body lotion in Miami but need a body cream in Aspen. Creams are also sometimes designed to follow body lotions for more in-depth treatment. Women will tend to use body creams more than men.

BODY OILS

Body oils may or may not be heavier than creams or lotions. Oils of late are being developed to be highly absorptive and function with a feel like oil but an absorption capability like lotion. Body oils are preferred to lotions by many with dry skin. Psychologically oils sound like they do more and soften skin better. This depends entirely on the specific formulation. But because the technology of oils has advanced so much in recent years, your clients should be buying them from you instead of using baby oil or cooking oil. You, once again, have the ability to specify the oil that's suitable.

Aromatherapy essences are very compatible with oils and work efficiently in oil bases. Men also generally prefer oils to creams or lotions as long as they aren't too greasy. Oils, if light, may also be used under a body cream for extra treatment. Spray-on type oils are highly popular today and are more common in professional products than grocery or drug store brands because the technology to make a great spray-on oil generally limits the oil to a finer grade substance. If you have a spray-on oil in your line, this is an automatic selling point that makes you different.

Specialty and Spot Treatments

This is the category in which you can really stand out and shine. All of the previously mentioned products compete in some form or another with over-the-counter brands, but this category often doesn't exist in over-the-counter form. This is the category in which you may find serums, liposomal lotions, ampoules, bust products, special splashes, cellulite creams, and so forth. Depending on your product line, you might want to call this group the treatment products, because they often are. The more sophisticated your day spa treatments, the more sophisticated your home care can and should be. After you have been able to gain the trust and product sales of the regular products, it's important to begin training your clients on the more serious treatment-based products.

SERUMS/AMPOULES

Serums and ampoules are normally highly concentrated active agents in a liquid or liposomal format to be used for special treatment of a specified condition. Normally serums or ampoules are applied at the end of a bath after all the cleansing and scrubbing processes are completed and just before the final moisturizing lotion, cream, or oil. Different products are used in different ways so you must look to your supplier for the specifics, but in general this is how they would be used. The specialty serum/ampoule probably has a very specific goal and works best with regular use daily over a period of time. This application and the duration must be specifically taught to clients and reviewed from time to time. A client will easily purchase this once but often it sits on the shelf unused for the most part due to ignorance or forgetfulness. You must actively control the usage to make it cost effective and results efficient for the client.

CELLULITE

For the ultimate in effectiveness in combatting cellulite, the client with this problem must be on a good regimen of treatment at home. Most product lines offer products to fight cellulite in the form of bath additives, treatment gels or lotions, and finishing creams. If all three products exist, the client should be using all three. If your line has only a bath additive and a cellulite cream, use both. Diligence and consistency is the name of the game in cellulite! The best way to make the most of these products is for the technician to confer with the client in person or by phone periodically between treatments to keep the client accountable and dedicated. But do so without badgering the client. Cellulite products should be sold in conjunction with a specific game plan at the spa and at home. This combination spells success! Basically only women get cellulite unless the man has a serious hormonal dysfunction, so this group is sold to women.

FIRMING CREAMS

Firming creams are designed to tone and firm the skin. They may be based upon proteins or aromatherapy to stimulate the skin and underlying tissues. As with cellulite, only regular, diligent use will make these effective. They are most often used by women.

BUST PRODUCTS

This is an interesting and growing group of serums, creams, sprays, lotions, and tonics. The reality of bust treatment at home is similar to cellulite. It will be effective only with dedication and regular usage. The effects that can be expected are smoother, firmer skin; some improvement in muscle tone; and overall improved texture. Bust products are obviously targeted for women but should not be used by lactating mothers. Sometimes stretch marks can be alleviated by usage throughout the pregnancy, not so much after.

MUSCLE PAIN RELIEF

Some of the aromatherapy ingredients such as menthol, camphor, and clove work well in lotions, liquids, and creams to relieve soreness and stress. Some product lines even have products with these ingredients to relieve tired legs and feet. The products can be in the format of serums, lotions, or creams and are a growing product category due to American lifestyles and the maturing of the baby boomers. Men will gravitate to these products for sure and so will working, career-based women.

OTHER

There are many other individual products such as water splashes, body finishing powders. All of these products are valuable to the day spa and should be integrated into the overall concept. Some are male oriented and some are more generic. Look to your suppliers for details on other products.

. . . .

SPA POINT

The specialty products are at first perhaps hard to sell but with experience and time will become the real builders of client ownership. These are the targeted products that you will know best and can own your client with. They are the items that fit a specific need and if they are good, will commit your clients to a richer, healthier life. They will also tie that client to the day spa concept and to all of your professional treatments.

. . . .

WATER FOR HOME USE

An interesting thought to facilitate the importance of product treatment along with bathing comes from research into the quality of water and potential contaminants in water today. According to a research project quoted in Encyclopedia Britannica's *Medical and Health Annual* (1991) "between 29 and 91% of organic solvents people are exposed to daily could enter the body during a 15 minute bath—substantially more than from drinking 2 liters (1 liter is slightly more than 1 quart) of water." So think of the nutrients that can also be absorbed by the body through bathing.

Hydrotherapy at Home

Hydrotherapy is a vital link to the success of a home-care program through the wonderful bath products and additives for improving well-being, softening and conditioning skin, and reducing cellulite. It's important, however, to consult with the client and develop a good understanding of what hydrotherapy at home really is, what bath additives to use, and how the client can help the in-spa treatment and home care goals that have been set.

. . . .

SPA POINT

In spite of the fact that we all know we can't live without water, we seldom consider the truly beneficial effects that water can provide. We tend to take this wonderful substance for granted.

. . . .

Baths and Showers at Home

Your clients don't need the detailed information you need on hot and cold water treatment but it might be helpful to briefly explain in simple terms what hot and cold water will do. Hot baths/showers calm, relax, sedate, and depress. This is good for bedtime. Cold baths/showers invigorate and increase tone and energy. This is good when you need to wake up or revive. Remember, cold for too long will reverse and depress, so cold baths should be short.

HOT BATH

Ideally this is done at the end of the day to relax, relieve tension, and allow bath essences or bath salts to further treat the body for whatever purpose is desired. Baths are probably the best mode of continued spa treatment at home depending on the additives.

There are a myriad of fine additives for the bath available from professional suppliers as well as from consumer retail establishments. It's important that you recommend the products for home use to prevent your client from buying elsewhere. Since the consumer tends to judge these products more from an esthetic viewpoint (look, fragrance, etc.), you should take control to make suggestions on the proper and most effective products to use. Remember, if clients are using bath products anyway, they might as well be purchasing them from you. Most additives provide instructions for use, but if that is not available, the typical length of time for a bath is normally about 20 minutes. If the bath water cools off too quickly, let some water out of the tub and add more hot water to maintain a comfortably warm temperature.

SOME PLEASANT BATH ADDITIVES

Again, professional products are recommended rather than home care remedies, but when professional products are unavailable, there are additives such as Epsom salts for muscle relaxation and perspiration stimulation. Apple cider vinegar is invigorating and if a lot (2-3 cups) is added to a bath, it's great to relieve itching. Sunburns are greatly relieved with 3-4 cups of oatmeal because the oatmeal tends to absorb the heat generated in the skin and may reduce some of the inflammation.

Professional products are, of course, better because they may do more for the body and they complete the spa program at home. Chamomile and lavender are great for relaxing; seaweeds and muds are great to mineralize the body; and essential oils like pine, rosemary, and clove are stimulating and help with elimination. (See chapter 6 on aromatherapy for more details.) Although the specific amount of the additive may differ between suppliers, as a general rule, add about 1-2 cups of the herbs, diluted oils, or salts to a full bathtub. If putting pure essential oils in a bath, the number of drops should range from 10 to 30 drops according to the essence.

HOT SHOWER

Showering is, of course, the quickest type of water therapy and probably the choice of most men and busy people. Most people consider a bath a luxurious thing to do periodically but shower daily or twice a day. The shower alone has benefits just from the water. But when combined with a brush or sponge massage, the circulation is revved up more and subsequent application of moisturizers and lotions penetrates better.

Even without any form of rubbing the shower alone can relax and yet stimulate the body and elicit a reviving response. That's why most people feel more awake and invigorated in the shower. Obviously a shower head that can be adjusted to different streams of water is good to provide a massage effect. Bath products to exfoliate or stimulate the skin can be applied before the shower and rinsed-penetrated in the shower. A quick hot shower is invigorating. A long hot shower will be relaxing and depressing to the body so it's best to take a quick shower in the morning and a long shower at night before bed, or a quick shower in the morning and a bath at night.

COLD BATH/SHOWER

Although it is rare to take a cold bath, it would be very invigorating to do so. However, another way to accomplish this is simply to take a quick cold shower. It's quite easy to switch from the hot water to cold water just at the end for a minute or two. The result will be a dramatically increased level of vigor. To take a cold shower after a warm shower is a typical Kneipp concept, and his belief was that this method of daily showering would go far to prolong one's lifespan. In addition to the invigoration, the cooling contracts the skin's pores and helps tone up the skin and underlying muscles.

FRICTION BATHS AND SHOWERS

Briefly mentioned previously, the use of a washcloth, sponge, loofah, or brush to rev up the circulation while bathing or showering goes far in stimulating the metabolism and circulation. A brisk friction massage of the area where cellulite appears (thighs, buttocks, abdomen, upper arms) is highly recommended to heighten the effects of any treatment or product application programmed for cellulite reduction. Obviously you don't want to rub the skin raw but a slight tingling and reddening effect works well for cellulite. For the rest of the body, a mild comfortable tingle or slight pink tone to the skin is fine and the person will feel highly invigorated after the bath or shower.

It's important to teach the client to approach this slowly and carefully. If you sell scrubs or other exfoliants, you will want to replace the friction rub with these products. It's also prudent to set up a time schedule for usage, perhaps combining friction rubs too. For example, have the client do the product exfoliant/scrub once or twice a week according to the manufacturer's recommendations and just do the friction rub a couple of times a week. Again, specific guidance should be obtained from your product manufacturers.

WATER TREADING

Another typical Kneipp water therapy was to do cold or warm water treading in the tub. This might even be considered a type of water exercise. Cold water treading appears to be more beneficial than warm or hot water. Cold water treading helps with leg cramping, poor circulation, overall exhaustion or weakness, aching feet and legs, and varicose veins. The idea is to fill the bathtub with enough cold water to reach the top of the ankles or even midcalf and then just walk in place (tread) for up to 5 minutes. Kneipp believed that this should be done daily for 2–5 minutes for the ultimate in invigorating treatment. This is an excellent treatment for anyone with circulatory or foot problems and really helps relieve discomfort. It's also an excellent way to get the day started. You may want to suggest a 5-minute cold water treading at the end of the shower or bath.

FOOT AND HAND BATHS

The hands and feet take the brunt of body punishment during the day and are therefore more exhausted than you might think. At the end of the day, a 5-minute cold or warm soak can have the effect of invigorating or relaxing the whole body respectively. This can be done with a foot bath, of course. Or you may use a shower massage device on a hose and just rain on the hands or feet for a few minutes. Or you may just put the hands or feet under running water from the faucet for the same amount of time. It's surprising how effective this is in restoring energy to the body.

TARGET SHOWERS

Sometimes directing the shower to a specific area of the body with warm or cold water will help relieve discomfort. For example, if the lower back is sore, it's good to target the shower for 3–5 minutes on the lower back area. To target warm water will relieve muscle soreness, but if the area is swollen, cold water is better. After a long day standing on your feet, you may want to do a treading foot bath, then target shower the lower back with cool water.

· ·

SPA POINT

There are any number of ways to use hot and cold water in baths and showers. In general warm to hot baths/showers relax and cold baths/showers invigorate. Short durations tend to invigorate and long durations tend to depress and relax the system. So a short cold shower is invigorating to get ready for the day. A long warm bath is relaxing at night and will facilitate sleep.

· ·

Compresses

We tend to think of compresses for ailments but certain compresses can also be beneficial for healthy persons. Warm or cool compresses may relieve fatigue or soreness or just add to the penetration of a cosmetic applied to the skin underneath. A hot compress will relax; a cold compress will stimulate and relieve swelling. Alternating hot and cold calms and stimulates alternatively. An interesting effect of a cold compress when covered by a dry cloth is that it heats. As the cold begins to wear off, heat generated under the skin causes a warming effect that will, in turn, stimulate circulation. Warm compresses when applied to the skin for a long period of time (15–20 minutes) are relaxing and soothing. A short cool compress (3–5 minutes) is stimulating. So sometimes when you want to increase skin absorption of a serum, ampoule, or lotion, a cool compress will stimulate the circulation for better penetration.

Cool compresses are also used when a person is bathing, particularly when taking a hot bath. Cool is better to use than cold, as sometimes a very cold compress on the forehead when bathing can cause a headache. Cool compresses will be used with professional hydrotherapy tub treatments as well as at home when taking a 15–30-minute bath. Compresses for health purposes may be infused with substances, but when using in conjunction with hydrotherapy it is recommended that the compress not contain additives. The additives in the compress can compete with additives in the tub. Just use plain water for the compresses.

· ·

SPA POINT

Even just plain water compresses when used locally can facilitate penetration of active substances for nutrition, can relieve stress and strain, and can calm or stimulate an area of the body.

· ·

Drinking Water

There is no question about the importance of drinking water. Without water the human organism cannot survive. Water quenches thirst, helps food dissolve, revitalizes internal organs, and helps improve elimination, to name just a few of its vital functions. The reality is, however, that most people don't think about the importance of water much less drink enough of it daily. When someone is ill or has a cold, what does the physician recommend first? That's right, drink lots of water and fluids. The purpose of this is to flush toxins from the system. If a person is prone to constipation, increased intake of water is believed to help relieve this problem as well, yet doesn't particularly cause the opposite to take place. The point to be made here is the value of water for overall proper functioning of the whole body.

It might be a good idea to investigate the quality of drinking water in your area so that you know if you should recommend bottled water. As a general rule, bottled water is normally healthier. There are now dozens if not hundreds of bottled water options from which to choose. Bottled water sales have increased more than 400 percent in the last decade alone, according to Encyclopedia Britannica's *Medical and Health Annual* (1991), which goes on to say, "one out of every 15 households use bottled water. In 1988 alone, Americans drank over 6 million liters of bottled water, a per capita consumption of about 24.3 liters." By the year 2000 we anticipate that this number will have drastically increased. Water is regulated as a food by the Food and Drug Administration (FDA), and there are criteria established for bottled waters as well as natural waters.

Although bottled mineral waters are often recommended, it should be remembered that they contain excessive amounts of minerals according to the FDA and as such, may not be recommended for total water consumption, although this is a controversial point. It's also controversial how much vitamin/mineral intake people should have, so consider your sources of regular water and drink mineral waters accordingly.

· ·

SPA POINT

Water is a critically valuable substance to maintain health and to facilitate the body's ability to increase metabolism and elimination, both of which will help in cellulite reduction, improved skin texture, and general well-being.

· ·

GENERAL BENEFITS OF INCREASED WATER CONSUMPTION

- Increases overall fluid flow in the body.

- Improves flow of blood and lymph, thus facilitating elimination of toxins.

- Stimulates kidney and liver to function more smoothly.

- Helps overcome constipation.

- Improves hydration level of the skin and internal organs.

- Helps keep skin more supple by maintaining moisture balance.

- The minerals in some mineral waters facilitate a sense of well-being and fight infections.

- Helps diabetics process sugars and helps to eliminate unoxidized sugars in the system.

- Salt in water helps athletes restore energy after excessive exercise and from loss of moisture through perspiration.

- Cool water may help reduce fever and help regulate internal body temperature.

SUGGESTIONS ON WATER DRINKING

- Make it a rule to drink at least six to eight 8-ounce glasses of water a day.

- Drink two glasses of cold water in the morning to invigorate the internal system.

- Drink a good blend of cold and hot liquids.

DRINKING OTHER LIQUIDS

Do not overdo consumption of coffee and other caffeinated drinks. Herbal teas are recommended for their aromatherapeutic effects as well as for sedative or stimulating effects. As an example, cinnamon or peppermint teas are great stimulants whereas chamomile teas are calming and relaxing. Relaxing teas are a nice complement to bathing and are highly recommended before bed.

Cellulite Treatment

Although cellulite treatment has been discussed from a number of angles, it should be kept in mind that any good cellulite program will include a dramatic increase in water drinking, friction massage in the bath, etc. The more hydrotherapy can be used with cellulite programs, the more effectively cellulite can be reduced. Drinking a lot of water alone will go far in helping to flush cellulite from the system. It's not a panacea, but it does help.

Synopsis

Water is a substance we all know we can't live without. What we often don't consider is the fact that water can greatly enhance our health and well-being. Water can help hydrate and soften skin, carry nutrients and essences into the skin, and relax or invigorate the entire organism. Water is probably the greatest spa therapy for professional as well as home use available to us. The key is targeting all the various forms of water treatment to the greatest advantage. And that's why the consumer needs you, the professional, and the day spa to maximize the great benefits there to be realized!

Home care is not only the solidifying factor for all the great treatments you'll do in the day spa, but also the money makers for you. A great technician is as strong at retail as in treatment for a very simple reason. You either believe in the whole concept, the ingredients, and the benefits or you don't. If you do, then you have a responsibility to try to manage the products your clients use at home. You must retail products to achieve the optimum benefits of ongoing spa treatment. And finally, from a purely business standpoint, you will make more money in retail long term than in service. And if you're ill, your sales go on, but your services don't. Please now refer to *Day Spa Operations* for all your business-based needs.

Review

1. Why is retailing products important?
2. Is there a difference between grocery store soap and professional soap?
3. Why are bath additives important?
4. What must be sold with a shower gel to make it efficient and cost effective?
5. What is the difference between a body lotion and a body cream?
6. How should cellulite products be used at home to be effective?
7. Why are specialty products valuable for a day spa to have?
8. Can a person live without water?
9. List some modalities of home water usage.
10. What is the difference between taking a hot shower and a cold shower?
11. How can additives be beneficial in a bath?
12. Why is it important to increase water consumption if you are on a cellulite reduction program?

Answers to Review Questions _____

CHAPTER 1

1. The term *spa* comes from the name of a small town, Spau, near Liège, in Belgium.

2. Germany is a very strong *"kur"*-concept country.

3. Spas in Europe are more cure (to cure an ailment) oriented whereas spas in America are more fitness and health oriented.

4. Resort spas are located on a resort or hotel property. Amenity spas are similar, but the spa is not normally considered an important profit center. And destination spas are located in a hotel environment, but the goal is for a spa program during the stay.

5. Spas and day spas are compatible because the day spa can be a good follow-up to the started destination spa program. Additionally day spas introduce the concept of a destination spa on a small-scale basis.

CHAPTER 2

1. History helps us understand the benefits of water therapy as not just a new invention. Water therapy has been used for health and well-being throughout the ages.

2. Hydrotherapy began probably thousands of years before Christ.

3. Hippocrates based many cures on the concept that drinking water alone was therapeutic as was mixing water with other modalities.

4. Sebastian Kneipp is famous today for water and herbal treatments. He was a priest who, in the 1800s, used water to cure his own health problems and then developed water-based healing therapies for others.

5. Plain water is a therapy. As an example, the morning shower wakes you up if nothing else, or a bath makes you relax at night before bed.

6. Bath additives can add and enhance water alone by having an aromatherapeutic effect on the body.

7. Warm and cool water can have opposite effects on the body. Warm water tends to increase circulation but relax. Cool water increases circulation as well, but if used for only a short time invigorates the body and stimulates energy.

CHAPTER 3

1. We know the Romans were famous for bathing by the documentation of the 1,352 public fountains, 13 aqueducts, 11 thermae, and 926 public baths.

2. Roy Jacuzzi invented a type of whirlpool tub that has practically become a generic word for whirlpools.

3. Balneotherapy is merely the use of baths for therapy whereas thalassotherapy is the use of seaweed.

4. Hydrotherapy tubs are special due to the targeted jets of air and water along with the underwater hose for massage.

5. Three typical contraindications to hydrotherapy would be systemic disease, high and low blood pressure, and pregnancy.

6. The ideal temperature range is 94–98 degrees F.

7. Underwater massage helps strengthen muscles, stimulates and helps to beak up cellulite deposits, and increases circulation.

8. The major categories are plain water, aromatherapy, and thalassotherapy.

9. Seaweeds used are Spirulina, Fucus, Chondrus, Corallina, Ascophyllum Nodosum, Chlorella, Macrocystis. (Any two of these is a correct answer.)

10. The essential oils are lavender, Clary sage, melissa, ylang ylang, bergamot, chamomile. (Any three of these is a correct answer.)

CHAPTER 4

1. A shower is the most basic hydrotherapy tool and is vital for cleansing as well as certain product removal.

2. A Swiss shower has targeted shower heads that pulsate and can be temperature variegated for various types of therapeutic treatments.

3. A Vichy shower can be a treatment by itself. However, it's better to do in conjunction with a mud, seaweed, or exfoliation treatment to maximize the benefits and time for both individually.

4. A steam shower/cabinet/room provides moist heat for the person who can't tolerate dry heat. It also offers a common modality of hydrotherapy that the consumer understands.

5. Many treatments work well in combination with a Vichy shower but particularly mud and salt glows.

6. A Scotch hose is a pressure hose, similar to a fireman's hose, designed to help break up cellulite, stimulate targeted areas of the body, and increase circulation.

7. Good sanitation is essential for the safety and protection of the client as well as the protection and preservation of the business.

CHAPTER 5

1. Touch has many effects on the body, but, if nothing else, it goes a long way to relax and reassure a client ensuring a more effective treatment.

2. Research has shown that the hemoglobin levels of both client and technician go up during massage, which in turn increases oxygen to the body and energizes both.

3. The Father of Modern Massage is Peter Henry Ling of Sweden.

4. Respectability was hard in coming to the United States due to the historic prevalence of prostitution and opportunists.

5. Some of the important effects of massage are overall increase in the blood circulation, improvement in metabolism, relief of muscle discomfort and fatigue, relaxation, and improvement of skin texture. (Any two of these is a correct answer.)

6. Client consultation is imperative before a treatment to know your limitations as well as to learn about areas that might be relieved by the massage.

7. Some common contraindications of massage are systemic disease, infection, inflammation, open wounds, diabetes, and any time in doubt.

8. Effleurage is the movement most used in conjunction with body treatments.

CHAPTER 6

1. Maurice Gattefosse is considered to have developed aromatherapy.

2. Plants have been used for more than four thousand years. An example from the Bible might be John 12:3 where it is stated that Mary anointed Jesus' feet during the last supper.

3. Jasmine is the king because it's expensive but so versatile, pleasant, relaxing, and soothing. The queen is rose, which is again very expensive but soothing, cleansing, and least toxic and also serves as an antidepressant.

4. A good blend for combination skin might be geranium, neroli, and ylang ylang.

5. Some of the contraindications of aromatherapy might be allergic reactions, systemic disease, rashes, pregnancy, inflammation, infection, and doubtful situations. (Any two of these is a correct answer.)

6. Aromatherapy is important in day spas because it is so well tested over the course of history and so much research has shown its effectiveness on the body.

CHAPTER 7

1. Shyness is absolutely an important consideration particularly with Americans.

2. The body is a much larger area than the face, and contraindications may have a more systemic effect.

3. Clients need to be assured that draping and good coverage will be done and that the only area exposed will be the area actually being worked on.

4. A dry room is not built to handle water. A wet room is normally tiled and drained purposely for water exposure.

5. No glass should be allowed in a treatment area except perhaps the bottles of essential oils, because of the danger of breakage.

6. A bed warmer is designed for a person to lie on top of whereas an electric blanket is a cover only.

7. Sometimes bath sheets are preferable to bath towels to give the client a sense of coverage and security.

CHAPTER 8

1. The technician must truly believe in the necessity and effectiveness of the body treatments and must experience them to be totally successful.

2. Common contraindications of body treatments include heart disease, systemic disease, pregnancy, open wounds, inflammation, infection, and doubtful situations.

3. A salt glow rub is a popular destination spa treatment and one that is well known to the general public.

4. Spa treatments can't cure cellulite but can help control it if the client is dedicated to the full program of treatment and home-care activities.

5. Full-body seaweed mask, full-body mud mask, herbal body wrap, paraffin body wrap, body massage, body facial, and tanning were all dicussed in this chapter.

6. Back, cellulite, and antistress are the most popular spot treatments.

7. Hydrotherapy greatly intensifies and enhances any individual body treatment.

CHAPTER 9

1. Exfoliate means to split into or give off scales, laminae, or body cells; come off in thin layers or scales.

2. Exfoliants are the first treatments to refresh the skin and ready the body for more absorbing elements of other subsequent treatments.

3. Overexfoliation can occur. It causes temporary skin thinning but eventually may cause the skin to thicken and become rather leathery.

4. Mechanical and dissolving are the two types of exfoliants.

5. Dissolving exfoliants are sometimes preferred when the abrasiveness of the mechanical ones is too strong.

CHAPTER 10

1. Mud is synonymous with spas.

2. Clay should not be used on clients with high blood pressure.

3. Kaolin is used for deep cleansing, drawing, and tightening.

4. Clay is used in esthetics for skin softening, mineralization, metabolic stimulation, and relaxation. (Any two of these is a correct answer.)

5. Clay should not be mixed in a metal bowl.

6. A Vichy shower is good with mud treatments.

7. Contraindications include high blood pressure, systemic disease, pregnancy, allergies, and doubtful situations. (Any one of these is a correct answer.)

CHAPTER 11

1. Seventy percent of the earth is water.

2. Minerals, the water in seawater, and the oxygen from seaweed are all beneficial substances for humans.

3. Algae are plants that normally grow in seawater or fresh water, at the edge of water, and on some trees and rocks.

4. Algae are used to soften skin; mineralize the body; provide vitamins, minerals, and antioxidants to the body; and help the body regulate itself. (Any two of these is a correct answer.)

5. There is a multitude of treatments that can be done with seaweed including full-body masks, bath treatments, spot treatments, and facial masks. (Any two of these is a correct answer.)

6. Contraindications to seaweed treatment include systemic diseases, high or low blood pressure, allergies to seaweed and iodine, and questionable issues. (Any one of these is a correct answer.)

CHAPTER 12

1. Spot treatments target specific areas commonly of concern to the client and can draw the client into other treatments.

2. Basically hand and foot spa treatments are the same as spa manicures and pedicures but without the soaking and nail care steps.

3. The main goals of cellulite treatments are to stimulate circulation to allow the body to help rid itself of the fat and toxins.

4. A back treatment is great to remove dead cell buildup, extract comedones and pustules, and condition the skin.

5. A spa facial is basically the same as a regular facial but with an added concentration on exfoliation, seaweed, and aromatherapy.

6. A sauna provides dry heat at about 175 degrees F and is an option for those who can't take warm moist heat. It induces perspiration and increases circulation.

CHAPTER 13

1. Retailing is critical to solidify the salon treatment, add effectiveness to treatment goals, and to hold the client to the salon.

2. Professional soaps should be less drying, more hydrating, and normally gentler than regular grocery store soaps.

3. Bath additives provide a mini salon treatment at home in the tub.

4. A sponge must be sold with a shower gel.

5. Lotions tend to be thinner and more readily absorbed by the skin than creams which are richer and more emollient for the drier skins and climates.

6. A hit-and-miss approach to cellulite treatment at home will not be effective. Products and routines must be done as directed for effectiveness.

7. Specialty products are important to lock that client into the spa, and they offer a targeted, specific goal-minded approach to treatment. They add an extra dimension of effectiveness.

8. No, a person can't live without water.

9. A therapeutic water modality for use at home might be showers and baths, compresses, and even drinking water.

10. Hot showers relax and sedate whereas cold showers excite, invigorate, and energize.

11. Since sitting in a bath is so conducive to product absorption, bath additives are excellent carriers of nutrients for the body.

12. Water will help increase the metabolism and elimination, and this in turn helps the body flush toxins from the system.

Bibliography

Abehsera, Michel. *The Healing Clay*. New York: Carol Publishing Group, Swan House Publishing, 1979.

Buchman, Dian Dincin. *The Complete Book of Water Therapy*. New Canaan, Conn.: Keats Publishing Inc., 1994.

Campion, Margaret Reid. *Adult Hydrotherapy, A Practical Approach*. Oxford and London: Heinemann Medical Books, 1990.

———. *Hydrotherapy in Pediatrics*. Oxford and London: Heinemann Medical Books, 1985.

Carr, N.G. and B.A. Whitton. *The Biology of Blue-Green Algae*. Berkeley, Calif.: University of California Press, 1973.

Chapman, V.J. *Seaweeds and Their Uses*. London: Methuen & Company, 1970. (In U.S., Barnes and Noble Inc.)

Croutier, Alev Lytle. *Taking The Waters, Spirit*Art*Sensuality*. New York: Abbeville Press Publishers, 1992.

Dextreit, Raymond. *Our Earth, Our Cure*. New York: Swan House Publishing, 1974, 1979.

Encyclopedia Britannica, vols. 1,5,8. Chicago: E. B. William Benton Publishers, 1984.

Encyclopedia Britannica, *Medical and Health Annual*. Chicago: E. B. William Benton Publishers, 1991.

Goldberg, Audrey Githa. *Massage for the Beauty Therapist*. London: William Heinemann Ltd., 1972.

Grilli, Peter. *The Japanese Bath*. Tokyo: Kodansha International Ltd., 1985.

Hennessy, T. Hartley. *Sun, Wind, and Rain, A History and Explanation of Hydrotherapy*. New York: Vantage Press, 1973.

Horay, Patrick, and David Harp. *Hot Water Therapy*. Oakland, Calif.: New Harbinger Publications Inc., 1991.

Kneipp, Sebastian. *The Kneipp Cure*. New York: The Nature Publishing Co., 1949.

Lavabre, Marcel. *Aromatherapy Workbook*. Rochester, Vt.: Healing Arts Press, 1990.

Lehmann, Justus F. *Therapeutic Heat and Cold*. Baltimore: Williams and Wilkins, 1990.

Rose, Jeanne. *The Aromatherapy Book, Applications and Inhalations*. Berkeley, Calif.: North Atlantic Books, 1992.

Round, F.E. *The Biology of the Algae.* New York: St. Martin's Press, 1965.

Ryman, Daniele. *The Aromatherapy Handbook.* Essex, England: Daniel Co. Ltd., 1984.

Ryrie, Charles Caldwell. *The Ryrie Study Bible, New American Standard Version.* Chicago: Moody Press, 1978.

Smalley, Gary and John Trent. *The Gift of the Blessing.* Nashville: Thomas Nelson Publishers, 1993.

Smith, Gilbert M. *The Fresh Water Algae of the United States.* New York: McGraw Hill Book Co., 1950.

Thrash, Agatha and Calvin. *Home Remedies.* Seale, Ala.: Thrash Publications, 1981.

Tiffany, Lewis Hanford and William Deering. *Algae, The Grass of Many Waters.* Springfield, Ill.: Charles C. Thomas, 1938, 1958.

Tisserand, Robert. *The Art of Aromatherapy.* New York: Inner Traditions Ltd., 1977.

Williams, Ruth. *The Road to Radiant Health.* Kennewisk, Wash.: Health Books, 1994.

Winter, Ruth. *A Consumer's Dictionary of Cosmetic Ingredients.* New York: Crown Publishers, 1989.

Further Reading

Among the many books and resources used for reference, the following may be of particular interest to the reader.

1. Kneipp, Sebastian. *The Kneipp Cure*. The Nature Publishing Co. 1949.

2. Chapman, V. J. *Seaweeds and Their Uses*. Methuen & Company, London England. (in USA Barnes and Noble), 1970.

3. Lavabre, Marcel. *Aromatherapy Workbook*. Healing Arts Press, Rochester, Vermont, 1990.

4. Tisserand, Robert. *The Art of Aromatherapy*. Inner Traditions Ltd., New York, 1977.

5. Rose, Jeanne. *The Aromatherapy Book, Applications & Inhalations*. North Atlantic Books, Berkeley, California. 1992.

6. Campion, Margaret Reid. *Adult Hydrotherapy, A Practical Approach*. Heinemann Medical Books, Oxford and London, England, 1990.

7. Croutier, Alev Lytle. *Taking The Waters, Spirit*Art*Sensuality*. Abbeville Press Publishers, New York. 1992.

8. Hess, Shelley. *SalonOvations' Guide to Aromatherapy*. Milady Publishing Company, New York, 1994.

9. Michalun, Natalia. *Milady's Skin Care and Cosmetic Ingredients Dictionary*. Milady Publishing Company, New York, 1994.

Glossary/Index

NOTE: Numbers followed by f indicate illustrations; numbers followed by t indicate tables.

Notes

Notes

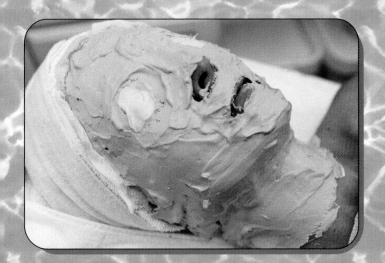

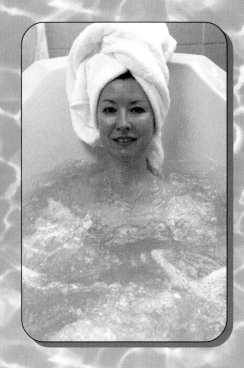

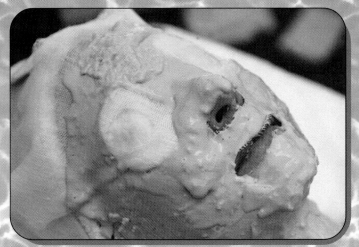

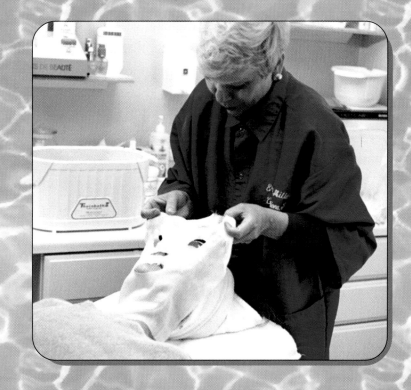

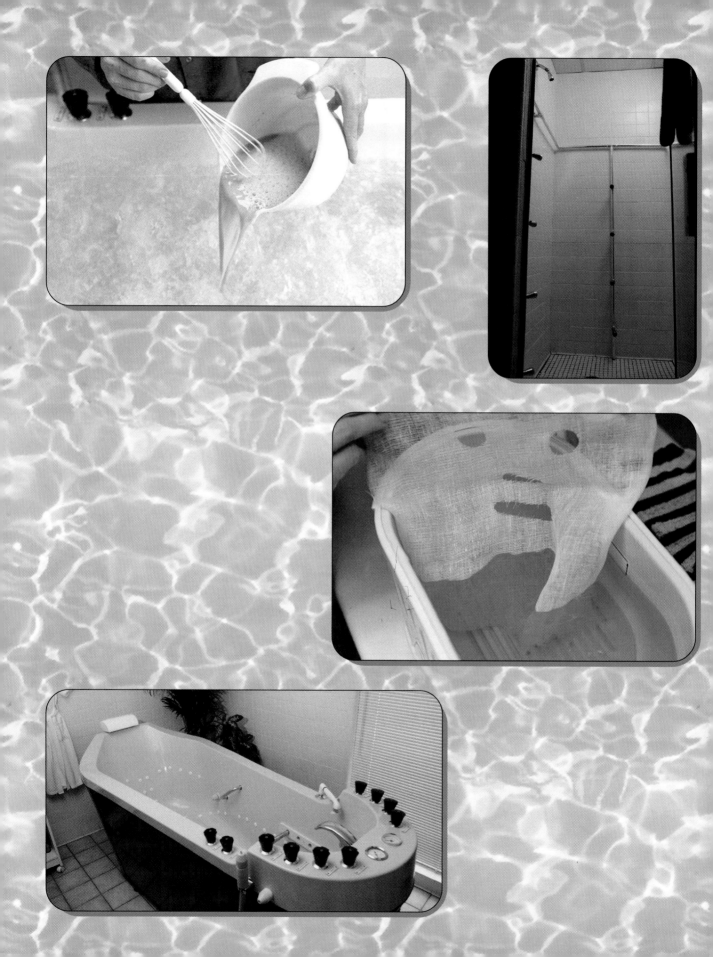

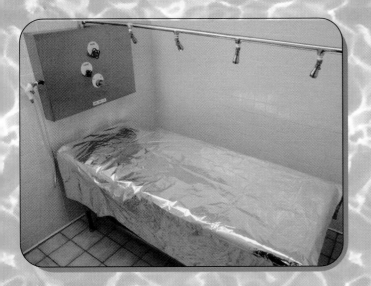

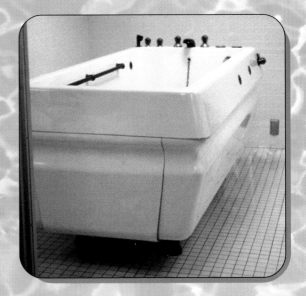

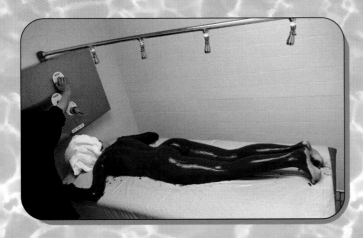

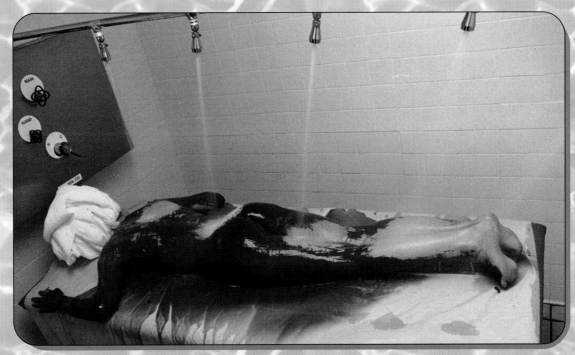

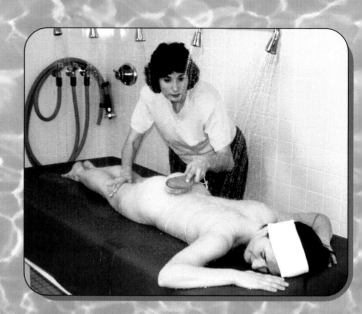

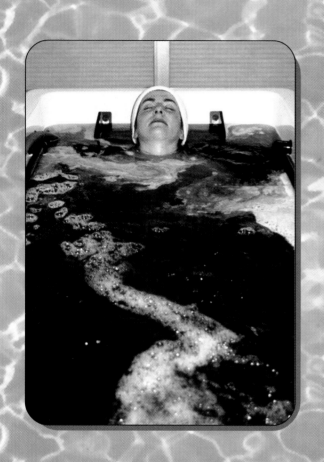

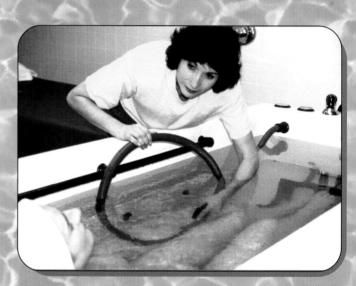

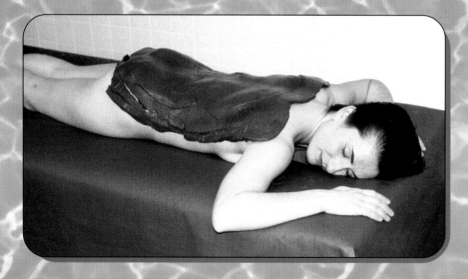